Reinvented

Your Midlife Blueprint to Balance Hormones, Boost Metabolism & Lose Body Fat — Naturally

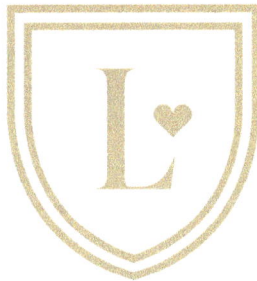

Copyright

Reinvented - Your Midlife Blueprint to Balance Hormones, Boost Metabolism & Lose Body Fat — Naturally

Disclaimer

The information provided in this book is for **educational and informational purposes only.** It is not intended as, and shall not be understood or construed as, **medical advice.**

While the authors, contributors, and publisher draw on current scientific research, personal experience, and professional expertise, we are not your personal physicians, dietitians, or healthcare providers. The content presented in this book is not a substitute for medical care, diagnosis, or treatment.

Before beginning any new diet, nutrition, exercise, or lifestyle program—including the strategies described in this book—you should consult your **physician or qualified healthcare professional** to ensure it is appropriate for your individual health circumstances.

Do not disregard professional medical advice or delay seeking it because of something you have read in this book. If you have or suspect you may have a medical condition, contact your doctor or other qualified health provider promptly.

The authors, contributors, and publisher expressly disclaim any liability for any adverse effects, injuries, or damages arising directly or indirectly from the use or application of any information contained in this book.

By reading this book, you acknowledge and agree that you are responsible for your own health decisions and that you will consult a healthcare professional before implementing any health-related program.

Table of Contents - Reinvented

Chapters

Chapters	Title	Page

Preface: When Doing Everything Right Still Isn't Working

Have you ever felt like you were doing everything *right* — eating clean, counting macros, tracking calories, following every bit of advice you could find — and yet, your body still refused to change?

That's exactly where I was.

For two years, I followed every rule I was told would lead to results. I committed to every plan, doubled down on my workouts, logged my meals, and stayed consistent. I tracked my macros, monitored my calories, fasted, and pushed harder at the gym.

And after all that effort? I lost just six pounds in two years.

Something inside me knew this wasn't about discipline. It was about biology.

I realized that most of the advice I had been following — from fasting to training intensity — was designed around how *men's* bodies work. Women are not men. Our hormones, muscles, and metabolism respond differently. What works for them doesn't always work for us, especially as we move through midlife and the hormonal shifts of perimenopause and menopause.

So I began to approach things differently. I stopped fighting my body and started listening to it.

I applied the framework that would eventually become the foundation of this book — a science-backed approach centered on glucose balance, hormone health, and strength preservation. And almost immediately, everything changed.

Within one month, I dropped **over 15lbs/6.8 kg of body fat and gained over 5% muscle mass.**
The same body that had plateaued for years finally responded — not because I pushed harder, but because I finally gave it what it needed.

I used tools like the **Withings Scale**, a glucose monitor device and **WHOOP** to track my progress — not to chase perfection, but to understand my body's rhythms and responses.

That experience changed how I see health, aging, and transformation.

Reinvented was born from that realization — that women deserve a framework designed for them: one that honors physiology, hormones, and strength.

This is not a diet book. It's not about restriction, punishment, or chasing a number on the scale. It's about learning how your body works, how to support it, and how to live in partnership with it — at every stage of life.

It took me two years to lose six pounds following conventional wisdom. It took one month to see real change when I began following *this* framework.

Now, I'm sharing it with you — so you can stop guessing, stop pushing, and start understanding.

Because your body isn't broken.
It's simply waiting for you to listen.

— Cho Phillips

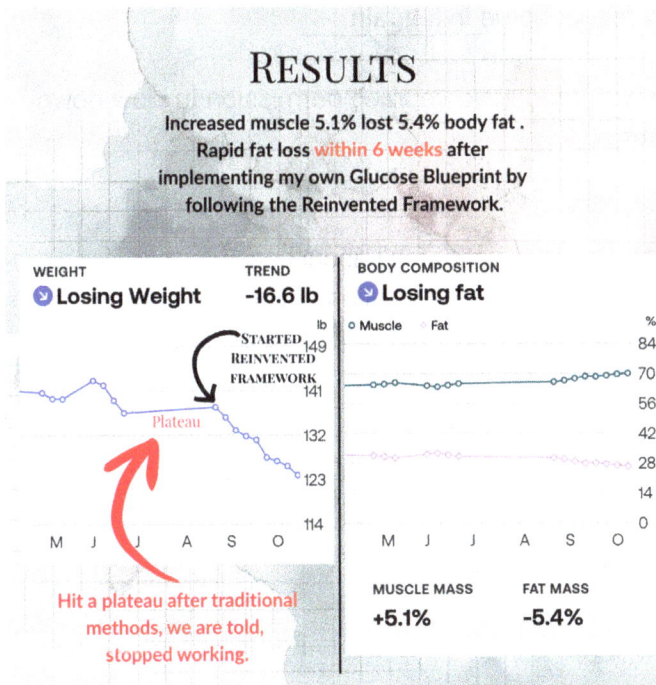

Author's Note

If you've ever felt stuck in a body that doesn't respond the way it used to, this book was written for you.

You are not alone, and you are not doing anything wrong. Your body is simply changing — and with the right understanding, those changes can become the very thing that sets you free.

The goal of *Reinvented* isn't just to help you lose weight. It's to help you rebuild trust with your body, learn its language, and finally feel at home in it again.

So as you read, give yourself permission to slow down.
To learn.
To listen.

Because transformation isn't about becoming someone new — it's about rediscovering the version of you that's always been there, waiting to feel strong, balanced, and alive.

Welcome to *Reinvented*.
Let's begin.

— Cho, Debra, Brooke

"Owning our story and loving ourselves through that process is the bravest thing that we'll ever do."

— Brené Brown

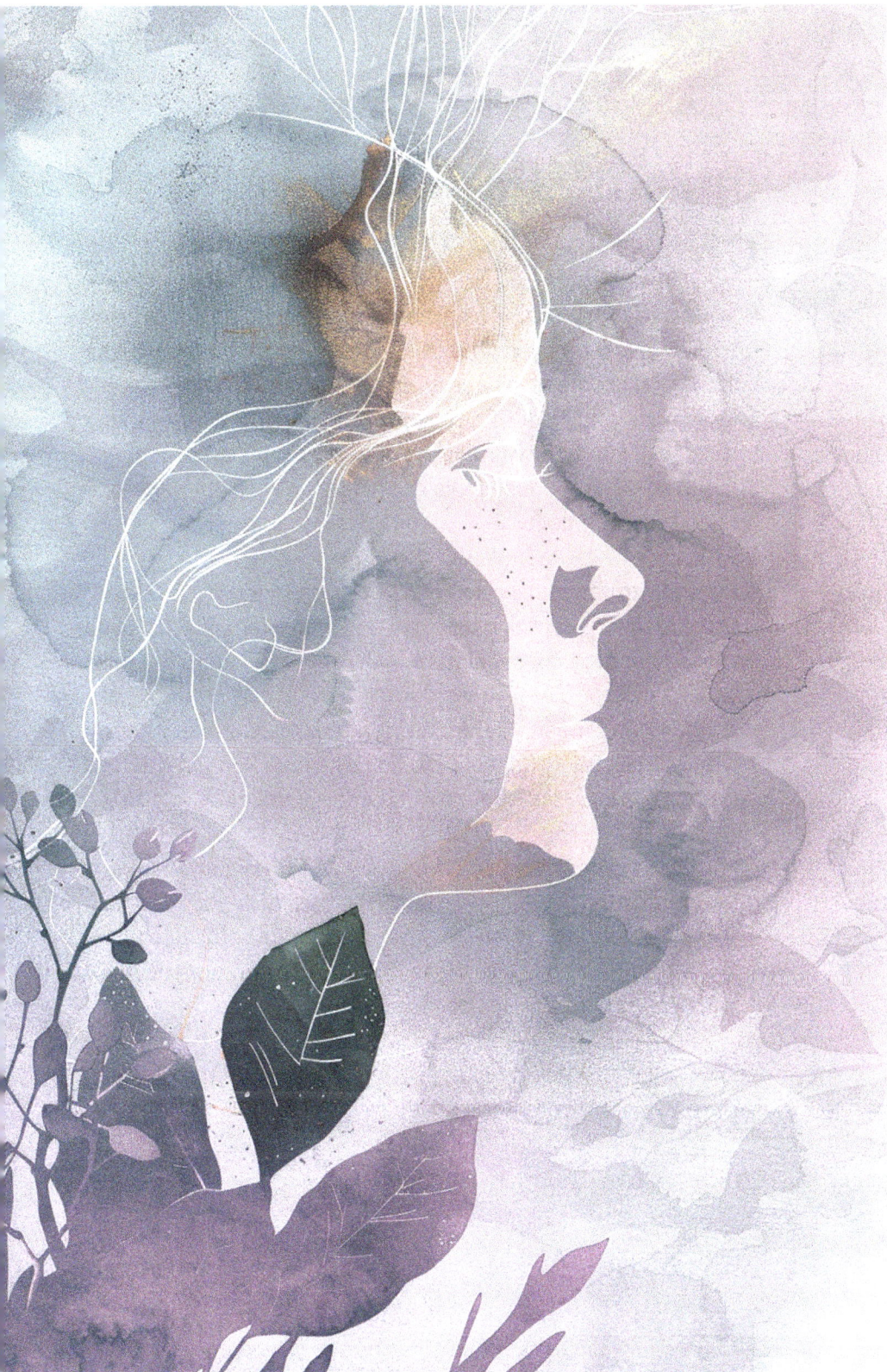

Introduction: A New Chapter for Your Body

If you're reading this book, chances are you've noticed that the rules you lived by in your 20s and 30s no longer apply. The pounds don't come off as easily, energy feels harder to come by, and despite your best efforts, your body seems to be working against you. For many women, the transition from perimenopause through post-menopause feels like hitting an invisible wall—one no one prepared us for.

Here's the truth: your body hasn't betrayed you. It's adapting. Hormonal shifts—declining estrogen and progesterone, fluctuating cortisol, changing thyroid signals—alter how you store fat, build muscle, and regulate energy. And while these changes are real, they don't mean you're destined for a slower metabolism, stubborn belly fat, or muscle loss. They mean you need a new playbook—one designed for this chapter of your life.

At the center of that playbook is one simple but powerful concept: **glucose control**. Glucose—the sugar that fuels your cells—is also the switch that determines whether your body stores fat, burns fat, or builds muscle. When glucose is well managed, your hormones work with you, not against you.

You'll have more energy, more stable moods, and the ability to reshape your body from the inside out.

Reinvented is about more than weight loss. It's about body transformation: losing fat while preserving—or even gaining—muscle, creating a metabolism that supports longevity, and building resilience for the decades ahead. The framework you'll learn here is grounded in research that focuses specifically on women, something that has been missing for far too long. For years, the majority of exercise and nutrition science came from studies on men. But you and I both know—we are not men. Our physiology is different, and our strategies should be, too.

You'll find science, yes, but also stories. Throughout these chapters, you'll meet women just like you: a 48-year-old suddenly struggling with midsection weight gain, a 52-year-old reversing prediabetes without medication, a 60-year-old rebuilding her bones with strength training. Their stories will remind you that you're not alone—and that change is possible at any age.

By the end of this book, you'll have the tools to design your own **Glucose Control Blueprint:** a personalized approach to eating, exercising, sleeping, and managing stress that keeps your blood sugar steady, your muscles strong, and your hormones in check. You'll know how to interpret your own body's signals, apply evidence-based strategies, and make adjustments that fit your lifestyle.

This isn't about quick fixes. It's about building a foundation for the next chapter of your life—one that's stronger, healthier, and more empowered than ever before.

So if you've ever thought, *"Something has changed, and I don't know how to fix it,"* this book is your answer. Let's rewrite the rules together.

A Note from the Authors: This Is Not a Diet Book

There are countless philosophies around food — Mediterranean, ketogenic, low-carb, plant-based, even carnivore — each claiming to be the solution. But the truth is, there's no single "right" diet for every woman. Our bodies, hormones, genetics, and lifestyles are beautifully unique. What fuels one woman's energy may drain another's.

Reinvented isn't about subscribing to a rigid plan or labeling foods as "good" or "bad." It's about understanding how your body responds to what you eat — and using that awareness to keep your glucose, energy, and metabolism balanced. The framework in this book teaches you how to listen to your biology so you can make empowered food choices that fit your life, your culture, and your goals.

This isn't about perfection or restriction — it's about precision and self-trust. When you learn how to work with your glucose, you gain the freedom to enjoy any style of eating, anywhere, with confidence.

"You are your best thing."

— Toni Morrison

How to Use This Book

This isn't a book you'll simply read and set aside. It's a guide, a playbook, and a workbook for your own transformation. Every chapter is designed to give you three things: **science you can trust, strategies you can apply, and stories that inspire you.**

Here's how to get the most out of it:

1. Follow the Framework, Step by Step

The book is organized in a way that mirrors the journey your body is going through. We'll start with understanding the hormonal shifts of perimenopause and post-menopause. Then we'll dive into the science of glucose and hormones, layer in exercise and nutrition, and build toward creating your own **Glucose Control Blueprint.** Each chapter builds on the one before, so take it in order—you'll see the full picture unfold.

2. Learn From the Stories

At the end of every chapter, you'll meet a woman who has walked this path. Their case studies aren't "before-and-after" gimmicks; they're real examples of women applying these strategies in different circumstances—struggling with prediabetes, navigating bone loss, or finding energy again after years of fatigue. Their wins (and setbacks) will help you see how to adapt these tools to your own life.

3. Engage With the Science Without Getting Lost in It

Throughout the book, you'll find references to studies that focus specifically on women. Science is powerful, but we'll always translate the data into plain language so you can understand what it means for you. You don't need to be a researcher—you just need to know how to apply the findings to your daily choices.

4. Use the Resources

At the back of the book, you'll find recipes, sample workouts, and tracking worksheets for glucose, nutrition, and strength. These aren't "rules" but tools—meant to help you customize your plan. You'll also find a summary of the key studies referenced, so if you're a curious reader, you can explore the research yourself.

5. Build *Your* Blueprint

This book isn't about copying someone else's plan. It's about creating your own. As you read, take notes, highlight strategies, and begin shaping a lifestyle that fits your schedule, your preferences, and your body's feedback. By the end, you'll have a personalized roadmap—your **Glucose Control Blueprint**—that you can use and adjust for years to come.

Pro tip: Don't just read—do. Try one strategy at a time. Track your progress. Notice how your body responds. This book is meant to live with you, in your kitchen, in the gym, and even on your nightstand as a reminder of what's possible.

Your transformation isn't about perfection; it's about progression. Every small step you take toward stabilizing your glucose, building muscle, and balancing hormones will create ripple effects in your health, energy, and confidence.

So grab a pen, keep your notes handy, and let's get started.

"Transformation begins the moment you stop chasing change and start choosing it."

Your Reinvention Begins Here

Before you turn the page into new habits, take a moment to pause.

This is the moment where awareness turns into intention. Before you dive into data and strategy, reconnect with the "why" behind your journey.

There are no wrong answers here, only quiet truths waiting to be rediscovered.

Reflect + Reinvent

1. What moments in your life made you realize something needed to change?

2. How have you defined "health" or "success" in the past, and how might that evolve now?

3. What limiting beliefs about your body, age, or metabolism are you ready to release?

4. What would it look like to feel completely at peace in your own skin?

5. What's one sentence that captures your personal definition of reinvention?

"The body is not an apology. It is not something to be fixed. It is beautiful, exactly as it is."

— Sonya Renee Taylor

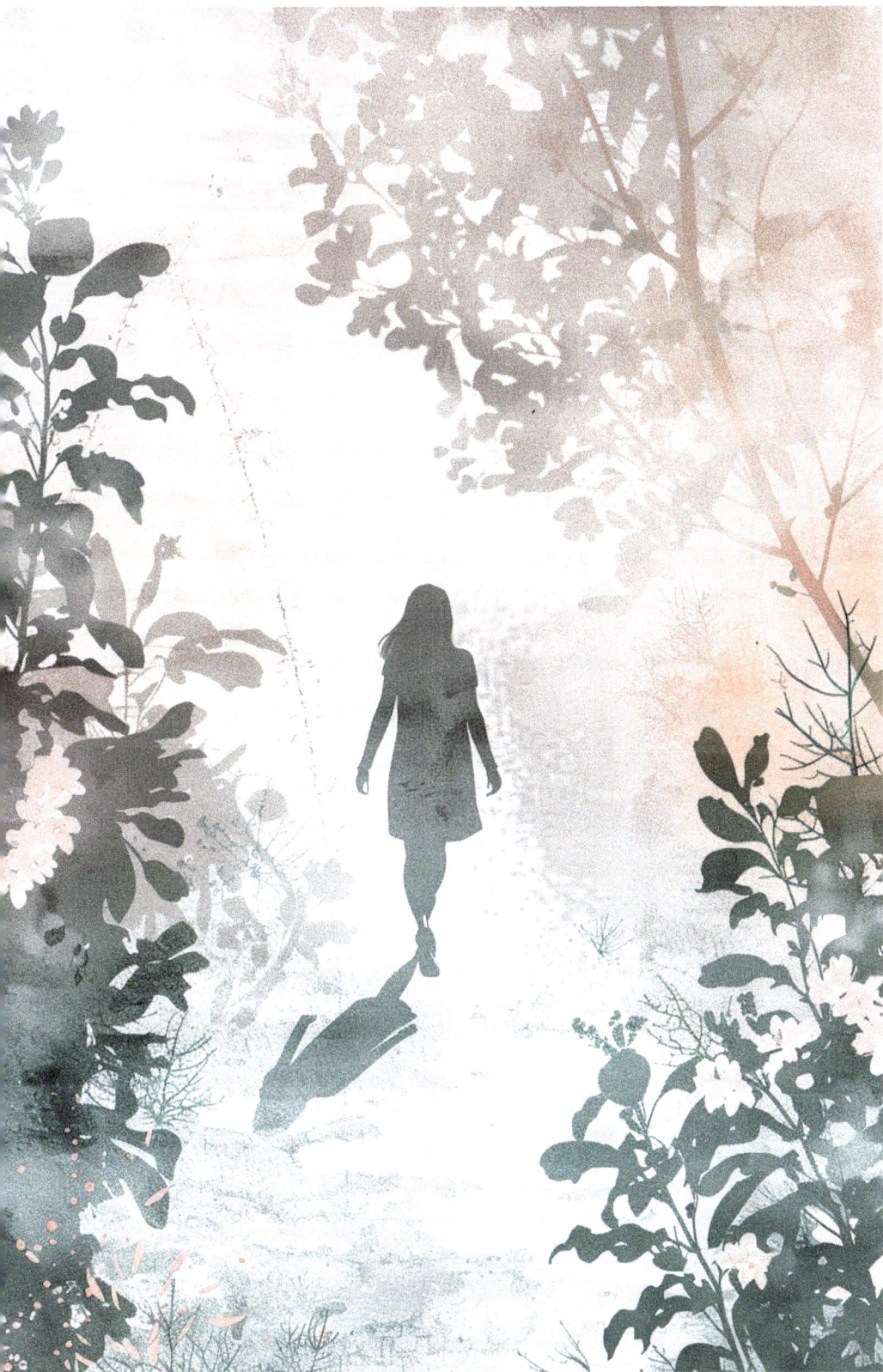

Chapter 1: The Midlife Body Reset — Why Perimenopause Through Post-Menopause is Different

If you've ever thought, *"My body feels like it's changed overnight,"* you're not alone. Many women in their 40s and 50s describe waking up one morning and realizing the strategies that used to work—cutting calories, adding a little extra cardio, skipping dessert—no longer deliver results. Suddenly, fat settles around the midsection, energy feels unpredictable, and workouts that used to feel empowering leave you drained. This is the midlife shift.

What's Really Happening Inside Your Body

Perimenopause marks the years leading up to menopause, when estrogen and progesterone production begins to fluctuate. These changes aren't linear—they can spike, dip, and rebound, which is why symptoms like hot flashes, irregular cycles, sleep disturbances, and weight gain can feel so unpredictable. Once menopause arrives (defined as 12 months without a period), estrogen and progesterone drop to consistently low levels, and the body settles into a new hormonal baseline.

Here's the key: estrogen isn't just about reproduction. It plays a vital role in regulating how your body stores fat, how sensitive your cells are to insulin, and how effectively you build and preserve muscle. With less estrogen, insulin resistance becomes more likely. That means the same meal that once fueled you smoothly can now trigger higher blood sugar spikes, stronger cravings, and increased fat storage—especially around the belly.

Cortisol, the stress hormone, also plays a larger role during this time. With disrupted sleep and changing hormone rhythms, cortisol levels often rise, further contributing to abdominal fat gain and glucose instability. Add in the natural slowing of thyroid activity and age-related muscle loss (sarcopenia), and you have a perfect storm that makes "traditional dieting" frustratingly ineffective.

Why Glucose Control is the Game-Changer

Most diet books talk about cutting calories or eliminating food groups, but few zoom in on the central lever: glucose. By stabilizing blood sugar, you improve insulin sensitivity, reduce fat storage signals, and regain access to fat as a fuel source. Glucose control is not about deprivation—it's about timing, food quality, exercise pairing, and lifestyle habits that work with your shifting physiology.

The good news? Research shows that women at every age—from perimenopause to post-menopause—can lose fat and gain or preserve muscle when glucose is managed properly alongside strength training and adequate protein intake. The days of starving yourself or running endless miles are over. This is about working smarter, not harder, and about tailoring strategies to your unique stage of life.

Case Study: Maria, 48 — "Why Am I Gaining Belly Fat All of a Sudden?"

Maria had always considered herself healthy. She wasn't obsessed with dieting, but she knew how to trim back when she wanted to lose a few pounds. Then, at 48, everything changed. Despite eating less and exercising more, she watched her waistline expand. She felt puffy, tired, and discouraged.

Her doctor reassured her that "this is normal at your age," but Maria wanted more than reassurance—she wanted a solution.

When she began tracking her glucose with a continuous monitor, she saw dramatic spikes after foods that never used to bother her—like her morning bagel or a glass of wine at dinner. By shifting her meals to include more protein, walking after dinner, and lifting weights twice a week, Maria began to lower her glucose numbers. Within months, her energy improved, cravings subsided, and her midsection fat began to shrink.

Maria's story highlights a critical truth: perimenopause isn't the end of your metabolic story—it's the beginning of a new chapter. With the right strategies, you can reset your body, stabilize your hormones, and move into post-menopause stronger, leaner, and more empowered than ever.

Chapter 1 Summary

Chapter Reflection: The Midlife Body Reset

As we close this chapter, one truth stands out: your body isn't broken — it's adapting.

You've learned that the shifts of perimenopause and post-menopause aren't punishments, but biological signals asking for new support. Estrogen and progesterone changes can alter how your body stores fat and processes glucose. Thyroid and cortisol step forward as key regulators, influencing how energized or depleted you feel.

These changes often make the "old rules" stop working — not because you've failed, but because those rules were never written for women's physiology in the first place.

What once worked in your 30s — cutting calories, doubling workouts, fasting harder — can now backfire, raising stress hormones and slowing results.

Here, you discovered that *glucose balance* is the foundation of midlife health. As estrogen declines, insulin sensitivity often follows. But by stabilizing blood sugar through mindful eating, muscle preservation, and recovery, you can reclaim energy, reduce fat gain, and rebuild strength where it matters most.

Maria's story reminded us that transformation begins with awareness. Her journey through frustration and plateau mirrors the experience of countless women who simply needed a new framework — not more willpower.

This chapter invited you to trade guilt for data, and exhaustion for strategy. The body you have today isn't the same one you had twenty years ago — and that's something to celebrate. It's wiser, more responsive, and ready for reinvention when you meet it with understanding instead of resistance.

Because the truth is: midlife isn't the beginning of decline — it's the beginning of precision.

The Shift — Redefining What's Possible

This chapter reframes the way we view women's health: not shrinking, but strengthening. Change often begins as discomfort — a whisper that the old way no longer fits. This is your moment to reframe what strength, beauty, and balance mean for you. Forget the rules written for someone else's body. These reflections are your permission to define wellness on your own terms.

Reflect + Reinvent

1. When was the last time you felt truly strong — physically, mentally, or emotionally?

2. What have you been taught about weight loss or aging that you now see differently?

3. How do you want to feel in your body six months from now — not just what you want to weigh?

4. What patterns or routines no longer serve your energy or well-being?

5. If "strong is the new steady," what does steady look like for you?

"Caring for myself is not self-indulgence, it is self-preservation."

— Audre Lorde

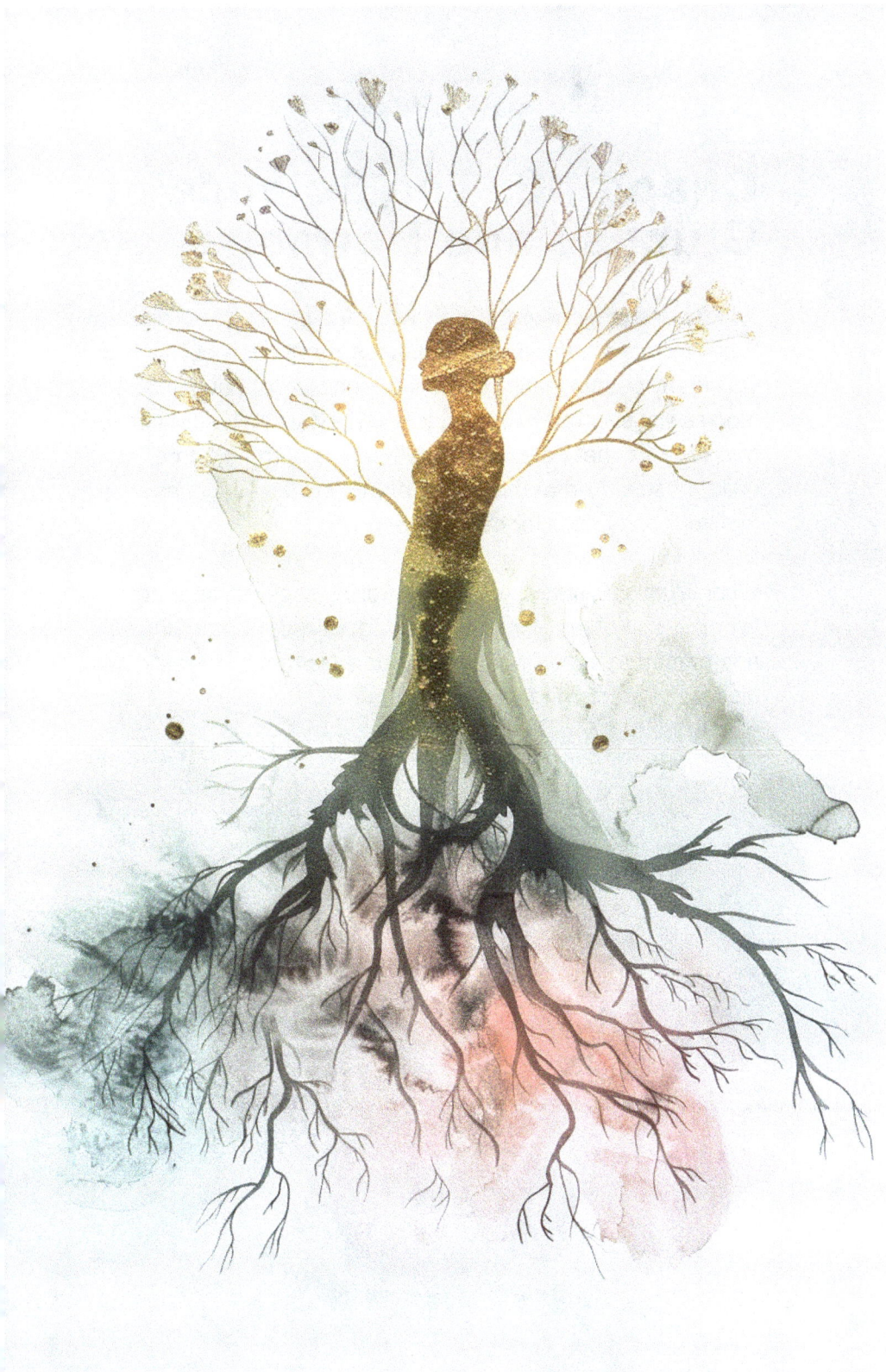

Chapter 2: The Science of Glucose and Hormones

You've probably heard the phrase, *"It's all about hormones."* When it comes to midlife body changes, that's true—but not in the way many people think. Hormones aren't just about hot flashes, mood swings, or reproductive cycles. They are powerful chemical messengers that determine whether you burn fat, store fat, or build muscle. And at the center of this system is glucose—the fuel your body uses for nearly everything.

When glucose is stable, you feel energized, focused, and satisfied. When it spikes and crashes, you feel tired, hungry, irritable, and primed to store fat. The good news is that by learning how glucose interacts with your key hormones, you gain back control of your body.

Meet Your Metabolic Cast of Characters

- **Insulin:** Think of insulin as the "traffic cop" for glucose. Its job is to move sugar out of your bloodstream and into your cells. But when insulin levels stay high (from frequent glucose spikes), your body stores more fat—especially in the belly. Women become more insulin resistant during and after menopause, which is why glucose control matters more now than ever.

- **Glucagon:** Insulin's opposite. When glucose is low, glucagon tells your body to release stored fuel and burn fat. In a well-balanced system, insulin and glucagon work like partners, keeping your metabolism flexible.

- **GLP-1 (Glucagon-Like Peptide-1):** You may recognize this hormone from the buzz around medications like Ozempic and Wegovy. GLP-1 slows digestion, helps you feel fuller longer, and lowers appetite—all while supporting glucose control. While medications harness GLP-1, lifestyle choices like protein-rich meals and fiber can naturally boost its effects.

- **Leptin & Ghrelin:** Leptin signals fullness, while ghrelin signals hunger. After weight loss, ghrelin tends to rise and leptin falls—one reason why it can be hard to maintain results. But glucose stability helps calm these fluctuations, making hunger signals easier to manage.

- **Cortisol:** The stress hormone. Chronically elevated cortisol raises glucose levels and makes belly fat harder to lose. Poor sleep and high stress keep cortisol high, which is why stress management isn't "optional" for body transformation—it's essential.

What the Research Shows

- Studies on women consistently show that even a **modest 5–10% weight loss** improves insulin sensitivity, lowers fasting glucose, and reduces fat storage signals.

- GLP-1 receptor agonists (like Ozempic) demonstrate how powerful glucose regulation can be, producing both weight loss and improved blood sugar control. But studies also show that **exercise, protein intake, and food timing** can mimic many of the same mechanisms naturally.

- Women who combine **resistance training with glucose-aware eating** maintain more lean mass during weight loss compared to diet alone.

- Lifestyle changes can even reverse prediabetes—improving glucose control and insulin sensitivity without major weight loss.

The takeaway? Glucose isn't just a number on a lab report. It's the central switch that determines whether your hormones are working with you or against you.

Case Study: Tanya, 52 — "Reversing Prediabetes Without Medication"

Tanya's annual checkup revealed something she feared: prediabetes. Her fasting glucose was creeping up, and her doctor warned she might need medication if it continued. Frustrated, Tanya wanted to take back control naturally.

She started by wearing a continuous glucose monitor for two weeks. What she discovered shocked her—her "healthy" morning smoothie (fruit juice, banana, and yogurt) sent her glucose soaring, leaving her tired and hungry by mid-morning. She swapped it for eggs and vegetables with avocado, and her glucose numbers lowered instantly.

By pairing her carbs with protein, walking for 10 minutes after meals, and adding two days of strength training per week, Tanya lowered her fasting glucose back to normal range within three months. She didn't just lose 12 pounds—she gained confidence that her body wasn't broken; it just needed a new approach.

Chapter 2 Summary

Chapter Reflection: The Science of Glucose and Hormones

If Chapter 1 helped you understand why midlife feels different, this chapter revealed how your body's chemistry responds — and how to finally work with it, not against it.

You learned that your metabolism isn't a mystery or a matter of willpower. It's an orchestra — one where hormones like insulin, glucagon, leptin, ghrelin, and GLP-1 each play a role in hunger, fullness, energy, and fat storage. When those instruments fall out of tune — as they often do in perimenopause and post-menopause — the result is fatigue, cravings, and that stubborn weight gain that seems to appear overnight.

But harmony is possible. This chapter showed that glucose regulation is the quiet conductor behind it all. When blood sugar stays steady, the rest of the hormonal symphony begins to play in rhythm again. Appetite calms. Energy stabilizes. Fat burning becomes effortless rather than forced.

You also discovered that medical tools like GLP-1 receptor agonists aren't magic — they simply mimic what your body can do naturally when supported by balanced meals, movement, and mindful recovery. Lifestyle can replicate the same benefits: slower digestion, greater fullness, fewer cravings, and sustainable energy — without dependency or side effects.

Tanya's story reminded us that it's never too late to turn your numbers — or your narrative — around. Her prediabetes reversal wasn't powered by pills, but by awareness. Each walk, each meal, each choice was a message to her metabolism: I'm on your side now.

The takeaway from this chapter is simple but profound — your hormones aren't the problem; they're the feedback. And when you nourish your body with consistency instead of restriction, it responds in kind — balancing, healing, and thriving.

Because the secret to midlife metabolism isn't control. It's conversation.

The Glucose Connection

Food is one of the most intimate relationships we have — with memory, comfort, and nourishment. These reflections invite you to listen to your body's feedback instead of outside noise. Here, you'll begin to recognize patterns in energy, cravings, and calm, and discover how balance tastes when it's personal.

Food is more than fuel — it's communication. Every bite sends your body a message.

Reflect + Reinvent

1. How do your meals affect your energy, focus, and mood throughout the day?

2. What foods make you feel balanced and nourished — and which leave you sluggish or craving more?

3. Have you ever noticed emotional triggers tied to when or how you eat?

4. How could pairing meals with movement become a natural rhythm instead of a "rule"?

5. What would it look like to eat in partnership with your biology, not against it?

"I love the fact that I can now say, I'm strong."

— Serena Williams

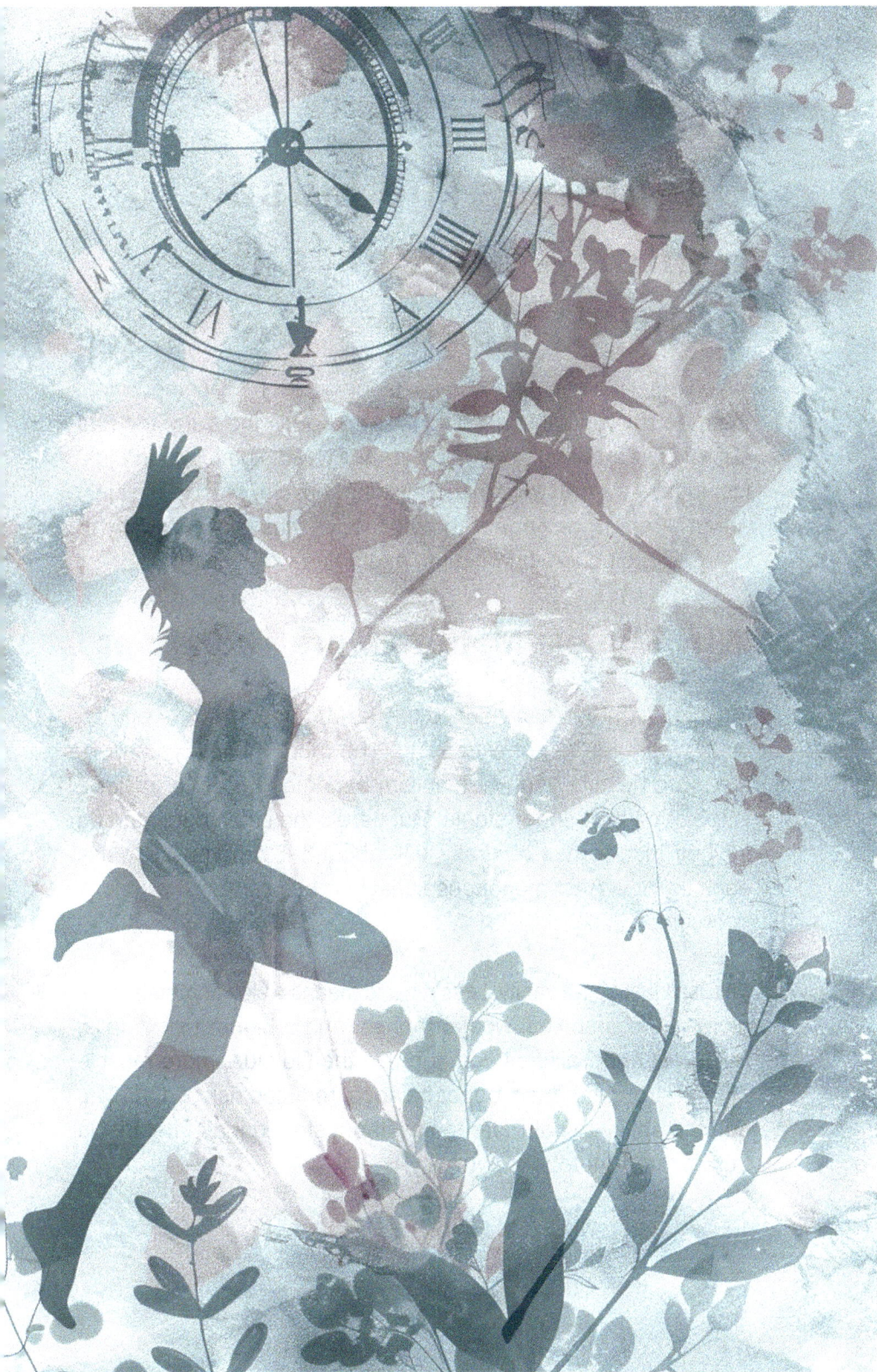

Chapter 3: The Muscle Factor — Preserve It, Build It, Use It

When most women think about changing their body composition, their focus is usually on losing fat. But here's the truth: the real secret to reshaping your body in midlife and beyond isn't just losing fat—it's preserving and building muscle. Muscle isn't just about strength or appearance; it's your most powerful ally in controlling glucose, burning fat, and aging well.

Why Muscle Matters More Than Ever

Muscle is metabolically active tissue—it burns glucose and fat even when you're not exercising. The more muscle you have, the more flexible your metabolism becomes, and the easier it is to keep blood sugar stable. But here's the challenge: starting in your 30s, women naturally lose about 3–5% of muscle mass each decade. After menopause, that loss accelerates if you don't intervene.

This isn't just about vanity. Less muscle means a slower metabolism, more glucose spikes, weaker bones, and a higher risk of falls, fractures, and frailty as you age. On the flip side, more muscle means stronger bones, better balance, reduced risk of diabetes, and the ability to eat more food without storing it as fat. Muscle truly is your "metabolic currency."

What the Research Says

The evidence is clear—and it's exciting:

- **Resistance training protects muscle during weight loss.** Studies show that women who only cut calories lose both fat and lean tissue, but those who add resistance training preserve, and sometimes even increase, muscle.

- **Strength gains are possible at every age.** In younger women, studies show rapid increases in lower-body strength—about 7% per week—when following progressive resistance training programs. In postmenopausal women, gains are slower but still significant, especially with higher-volume programs.

- **Muscle supports glucose control.** Resistance training improves insulin sensitivity and lowers fasting glucose, independent of weight loss. That means even before the scale moves, your metabolism is already improving.

- **Bone health improves with lifting.** Weight training doesn't just build muscle—it stimulates bone density, protecting against osteoporosis, which becomes more common after menopause.

The bottom line: if you're not lifting, you're leaving one of your most powerful fat-loss and longevity tools on the table.

How to Get Started

You don't need to live in the gym or lift like a bodybuilder to see results. Research shows that **2–3 days of resistance training per week** is enough to build strength, improve glucose control, and preserve lean mass during weight loss. Focus on compound movements—squats, deadlifts, rows, presses—that work multiple muscles at once. Pair strength training with adequate protein (at least 25–30 grams per meal) to maximize muscle repair and growth.

Think of muscle as the *container* that holds your transformation. Without it, fat loss is temporary and fragile. With it, fat loss becomes sustainable and empowering.

Case Study: Janet, 55 — "Strong, Lean, and Living Proof"

Janet had tried every diet out there. She could always lose a few pounds, but the weight crept back, and she felt weaker each time. At 55, frustrated by her "yo-yo" pattern, she joined a small-group strength training class. At first, she worried she was "too old" and "too out of shape" to lift weights. But within weeks, she noticed she was sleeping better, her cravings diminished, and her clothes fit differently—even though the scale barely moved.

Over six months, Janet lost 30 pounds of fat and gained noticeable muscle definition. More importantly, her glucose numbers improved, her doctor reduced her blood pressure medication, and she felt confident in her body again. Janet's story shows what the science makes clear: muscle changes everything.

Chapter 3 Summary

Chapter Reflection: The Muscle Factor — Preserve It, Build It, Use It

By now, you've begun to see your body not as a project to be fixed, but as a system to be understood — and nothing demonstrates that better than muscle.

In this chapter, you learned that muscle isn't just about tone or appearance — it's your body's most metabolically active tissue, a silent engine that burns glucose, supports bones, regulates hormones, and safeguards your longevity. It's not simply about looking strong; it's about *living* strong.

You saw how research redefines aging for women. Resistance training — once considered "optional" — is now recognized as essential medicine. Studies show that women can increase lower-body strength by as much as 7% per week when training consistently, and post-menopausal women still experience measurable gains in muscle and metabolism. The message? It's never too late. In fact, it's often the perfect time.

Janet's story brought this truth to life. At 55, she didn't just lose 30 pounds — she rebuilt her body from the inside out. Her transformation wasn't measured by the scale, but by strength, confidence, and vitality.

Muscle is metabolic gold. Every rep, every stretch, every mindful movement you make isn't just exercise — it's a conversation with your biology, reminding it to stay alive, active, and responsive. The real takeaway from this chapter is simple: when you build muscle, you build resilience. You teach your body how to stay strong through hormonal shifts, how to burn glucose efficiently, and how to age with grace — not fragility.

So the next time you lift, remember: you're not just shaping your body — you're shaping your future.

"Strong women aren't born; they're built — rep by rep, choice by choice."

The Muscle Factor

Muscle is more than tone or shape — it's a metabolic organ, your body's energy engine. It's not just a physical force — it's emotional architecture. Every time you lift, stretch, or move, you're not just sculpting your body; you're reshaping your relationship with resilience. Let these questions help you reconnect to your power — the kind that lives in both movement and stillness.

Reflect + Reinvent

1. What's your current relationship with strength training — joy, intimidation, avoidance, or empowerment?

2. How does movement affect your mood, confidence, and sense of control?

3. What would it mean to train for longevity, not aesthetics?

4. How can you build consistency in movement that feels natural, not forced?

If your muscles could talk, what would they thank you for?

"A woman is the full circle. Within her is the power to create, nurture, and transform."

— Diane Mariechild

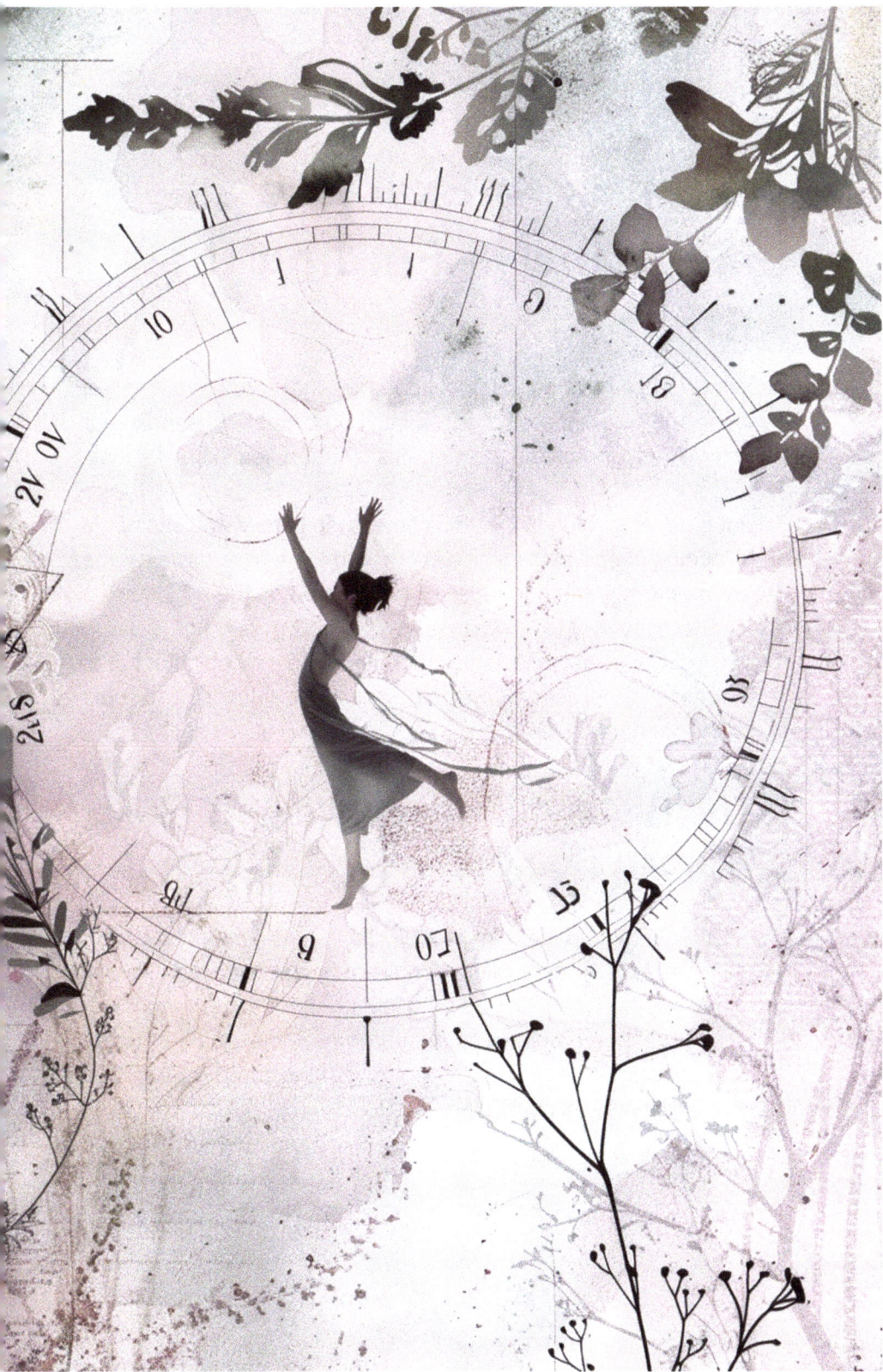

Chapter 4: Exercise as Medicine — Finding the Right Mix

Most women have been told for decades that cardio is the secret to weight loss. "Hop on the treadmill, burn calories, shrink your body." And yes—cardio has benefits for heart health and fat loss.

But the real revolution in midlife fitness isn't about endless hours of jogging or spin classes. It's about learning how to *use exercise like medicine*—the right dose, the right type, at the right time.

The goal? Not just to lose weight, but to create a body that burns fat efficiently, preserves muscle, regulates glucose, and feels strong for decades to come.

The Big Myth: Heavy Weights Make Women Bulky

Let's clear this up once and for all: lifting heavy weights will *not* make you bulky. Women simply don't produce enough testosterone to develop bodybuilder-sized muscles without extreme training, supplementation, and nutrition strategies. What heavy weights do is increase muscle strength, improve bone density, and shape your body in ways cardio never can.

Here's the distinction most people miss:

- **Hypertrophy (muscle growth)** happens when you train with moderate to heavy weights for multiple sets and reps (usually 6–12 reps, 3–5 sets). Over time, this builds muscle size and definition.

- **Maximal Strength (tone without bulk)** comes from lifting heavier weights for very few reps—sometimes even just one rep to *failure*—with 100% effort. This kind of training signals your nervous system to get stronger without necessarily adding muscle mass. The result? Firm, toned muscles without "bulking."

For example, doing 3 sets of 10 squats with increasing weight builds muscle size (hypertrophy). But pushing yourself to perform *one single pull-up* with maximum effort—or using negative reps to build toward that goal—builds raw strength, neurological adaptation, and visible tone without enlarging the muscle.

Myth Buster: Heavy Weights = Bulky Muscles

Nope. Women don't have the testosterone levels required to build massive muscle without extreme effort, specialized nutrition, or drugs. What heavy weights do is build strength, shape, and tone while burning more calories at rest. Translation: lifting heavy makes you leaner, not bulkier.

Tone vs. Bulk: What's the Difference?

- **Hypertrophy (bulk/size):** Moderate-to-heavy weights, 6–12 reps, multiple sets, consistent overload.
- **Strength (tone):** Very heavy weights or full-effort calisthenics (like one hard push-up or pull-up), low reps—even just 1—with 100% effort.

Tone = neurological strength + muscle firmness. Bulk = muscle growth + size.

Calisthenics: Proof That You Don't Need a Gym

If weights feel intimidating, calisthenics (bodyweight strength training) is an incredible entry point. Think of exercises like push-ups, pull-ups, squats, and planks. The magic here is not in endless reps, but in working toward a single, powerful goal.

Imagine setting the goal: "I want to do one proper push-up." Even if you can't do one yet, you start with negatives (lowering slowly to the floor), incline push-ups, and progressions that move you closer each week. Each rep is maximal effort, teaching your body to recruit more muscle fibers and build strength. The same applies to a pull-up goal. The training is simple, efficient, and doesn't require hours in the gym—just consistency and intensity.

This is where effort matters more than time. You can make incredible strength gains in short sessions (even one or two exercises done to true failure), if you're giving your body 100%.

Calisthenics = Freedom Fitness

No equipment? No problem. Push-ups, pull-ups, squats, lunges, planks, and dips are all you need. Training toward one challenging move (like a pull-up) builds strength and body control while torching fat and stabilizing glucose.

The Push-Up Blueprint

Goal: Do 1 proper push-up.
- Start with incline push-ups.
- Add negatives (lowering slowly).
- Progress week by week.

By training for just one rep at 100% effort, you'll build strength, tone, and confidence—without needing endless gym time.

Finding Your Exercise Prescription

Research on women shows clear patterns:

- **Aerobic exercise** is best for fat loss, heart health, and overall endurance.

- **Resistance training** is the gold standard for building and preserving muscle, improving glucose control, and preventing age-related decline.

- **The combination** delivers the most powerful body composition changes: fat down, muscle up.

The prescription isn't "spend hours in the gym." It's **2–3 strength sessions per week** (weights or calisthenics), plus 2–3 cardio sessions (walking, cycling, or anything you enjoy). Mix and match based on your lifestyle, and you'll cover all the bases.

Case Study: Lucy, 60 — "Stronger Bones, Stronger Body"

Lucy was terrified of lifting weights. She worried it would make her bulky and thought cardio was enough. But when a bone density scan revealed early osteoporosis, her doctor suggested resistance training. Reluctantly, Lucy began with light weights and bodyweight exercises.

At first, she couldn't do a single push-up. But by focusing on negatives, and then practicing one full-effort push-up attempt per workout, she slowly built strength. Over time, she added squats, rows, and overhead presses. Six months later, not only could Lucy do multiple push-ups, but her bone density had improved, her waistline was smaller, and she felt more confident than ever.

Her story illustrates the power of effort over time: even a few focused strength sessions per week created results she never thought possible.

You Can't Outrun a Donut

Cardio burns calories in the moment, but it doesn't offset poor glucose control. A 30-minute jog might burn ~250 calories, but one donut can spike glucose, raise insulin, and shut down fat burning for hours.

Strength training + glucose-stabilizing meals = longer-term fat loss.

Less is More with HIIT

HIIT works because of intensity, not duration. 2 sessions per week, 10–15 minutes each, with 2–5 intervals, is enough to boost insulin sensitivity, improve heart health, and torch fat. More than that can stress hormones.

Sprint, cycle, row, or even power walk uphill—just give 100% in short bursts.

DID YOU KNOW?

Why Strength Training Beats Cardio Alone

- **Cardio:** Best for fat loss and heart health.

- **Strength:** Best for muscle, glucose, and metabolism.

- **Combo:** The gold standard for women over 40.

If you only have time for one? Choose strength. It protects your metabolism for life.

HIIT — The 15-Minute Game Changer

Think you need to spend an hour on the treadmill to see results? Think again. Research shows that short bursts of high-intensity interval training (HIIT) can deliver outsized benefits for women in midlife and beyond—improving glucose control, fat loss, cardiovascular health, and even insulin sensitivity.

Here's how to do it:

- **Frequency:** 2 times per week is plenty.

- **Duration:** 10–15 minutes total.

- **Structure:** 2–5 intervals of "all-out" effort, lasting 30–60 seconds each, followed by full recovery.

Example HIIT Workout (10 minutes):

- Warm up for 3 minutes (walk, cycle, row).

- Sprint for 30 seconds (all out).

- Recover for 2 minutes (slow pace).

- Repeat 3 times.

- Cool down for 2 minutes.

That's it. In just 10 minutes, you've improved glucose uptake, boosted your metabolism, and reaped the benefits of a much longer cardio session.

Why it works: HIIT creates powerful adaptations without draining your energy or stressing your hormones like chronic cardio can. It trains your muscles to become more glucose-hungry and insulin-sensitive, making it a perfect complement to resistance training.

Pair HIIT with 2–3 strength sessions per week, and you've got a complete, time-efficient blueprint for fat loss and muscle preservation.

The Science of Confidence

Confidence isn't built in your mind first — it's built in your muscles. Every rep, every walk, every act of showing up for yourself sends a powerful message from your body to your brain: I can.

That message rewires your neurology — literally. Consistent physical activity increases dopamine receptor sensitivity, enhances prefrontal cortex activation (your decision-making center), and decreases amygdala reactivity (your stress center). Translation: movement builds mental resilience.

As muscle grows, metabolism rises. As metabolism strengthens, energy stabilizes. As energy steadies, your self-trust deepens — and that's where confidence lives.

Confidence isn't the absence of doubt; it's the presence of evidence. And your body keeps the receipts.

Each time you lift, stretch, breathe, or simply keep a promise to yourself, you reinforce a loop of empowerment. The woman who once questioned her strength now moves through life with it.

Science calls it adaptive capacity.

You'll feel it as self-trust — the quiet knowing that you are capable, powerful, and unshakably alive.

"Confidence is the chemistry of consistency — and your body is the lab."

Chapter 4 Summary

Chapter Reflection: Exercise as Medicine — The Power of Movement

If food is information, then movement is medicine — and this chapter reminded us that how we move determines how we age.

You learned that not all exercise serves the same purpose. Resistance training builds and preserves muscle — the very tissue that fuels your metabolism and stabilizes glucose. Aerobic activity, meanwhile, trims fat, strengthens the heart, and enhances oxygen efficiency. But when you combine the two — strength and stamina — your body becomes a masterpiece of balance and adaptability.

The research couldn't be clearer: women who integrate both forms of movement experience the most dramatic improvements in body composition, cardiovascular health, and energy levels. Aerobic exercise may slim the silhouette, but resistance training sculpts the architecture beneath it — building shape, strength, and stability.

You also discovered that exercise isn't about doing more — it's about doing *better*. Overtraining or chasing endless cardio sessions can elevate cortisol and slow results, while strategic training builds a body that thrives. The goal is harmony — not exhaustion.

Lucy's story brought this science to life. At 60, lifting weights didn't just transform her muscle tone — it reversed bone loss and reignited confidence she hadn't felt in decades. Her journey proved that exercise isn't punishment for what we eat, but a privilege that teaches the body how to regenerate.

So as you move forward, remember this: every walk, lift, stretch, or climb sends a message to your body that you intend to keep living fully — strong, mobile, and radiant.

Exercise isn't just how we change our bodies. It's how we honor them.

The Movement Blueprint

Movement is a love language between your body and your mind. It doesn't have to be perfect — it just has to be yours.

Reflect + Reinvent

1. What types of movement feel good in your body right now?

2. How do you want movement to fit into your lifestyle — ritual, release, or recreation?

3. What's one limiting story you've told yourself about exercise that you're ready to rewrite?

4. What's the difference between discipline and devotion in how you move?

5. How can you bring more play into your physical routine?

"Move not to change your body — but to remember how powerful it already is."

"You don't have to cook fancy or complicated masterpieces— just good food from fresh ingredients."

— Julia Child

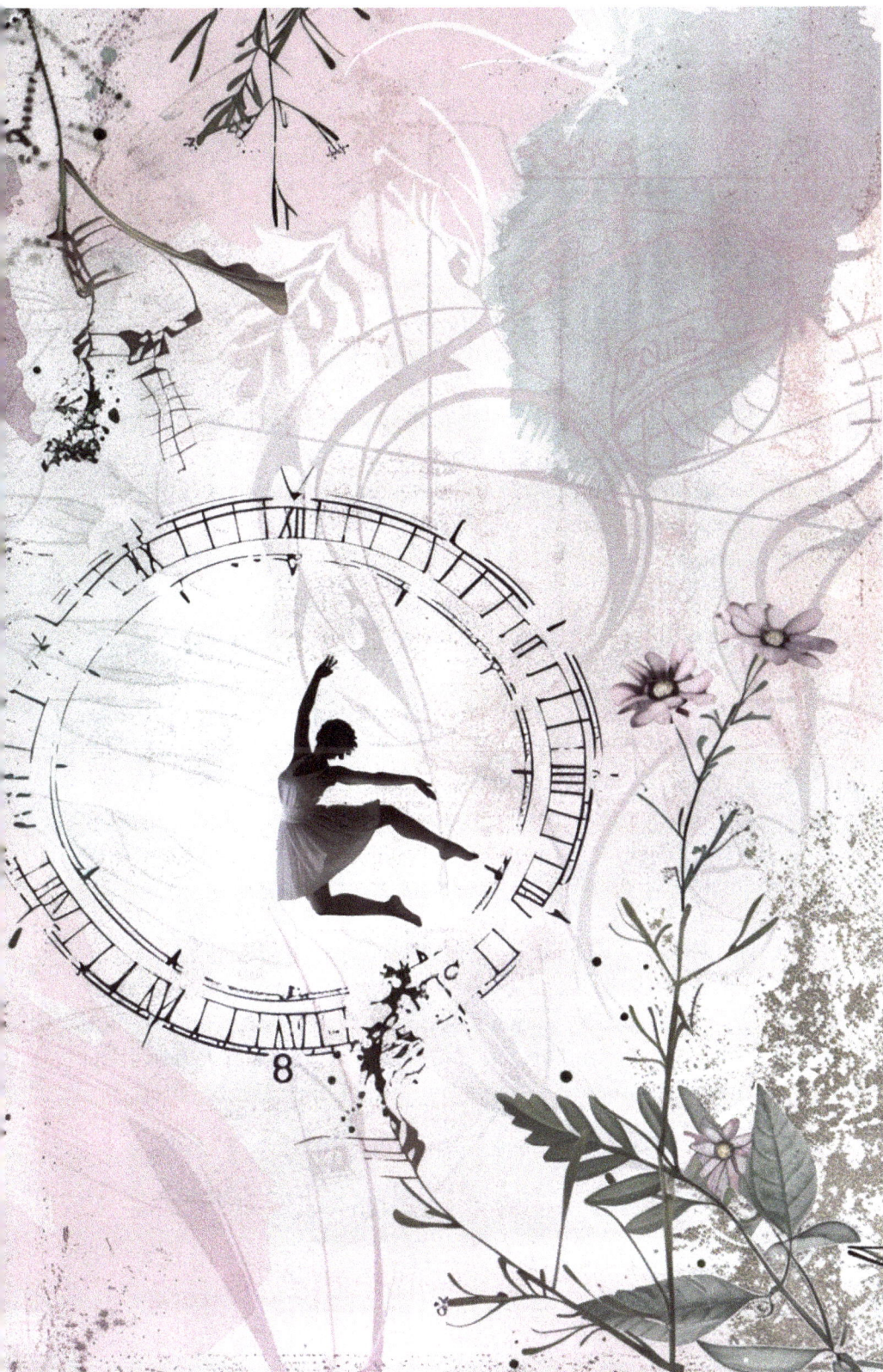

Chapter 5: Nutrition for Hormone Balance and Glucose Control

"You can't out-train a poor diet." You've probably heard that phrase before, and in midlife it becomes truer than ever. While exercise is crucial for building muscle and improving insulin sensitivity, what you put on your plate determines whether your glucose stays steady—or swings wildly, pulling your hormones along for the ride.

The Glucose–Food Connection

Here's the science in plain English: when you eat carbohydrates, they break down into glucose. Your body uses insulin to shuttle that glucose into your cells for energy. But when carbs are eaten alone, in large amounts, or as refined sugars, glucose spikes hard. Insulin follows, often overshooting, and the result is a crash—hunger, fatigue, cravings, and fat storage.

But when you eat carbs alongside protein, healthy fats, and fiber, the glucose rise is slower and smaller. Insulin doesn't surge as high, your energy stays steady, and your body can continue burning fat instead of storing it. This is why nutrition is less about elimination and more about **pairing, timing, and balance.**

Protein: Your Midlife Powerhouse

Protein isn't just for bodybuilders—it's the anchor of a midlife woman's diet. Why?

- It blunts glucose spikes.

- It supports muscle repair and growth after strength training.

- It increases satiety, so you feel fuller for longer.

Studies consistently show that women who eat **25–30 grams of protein** per meal preserve more lean mass during weight loss and maintain stronger bones post-menopause. Protein quality matters too—lean meats, fish, eggs, dairy, and plant proteins like lentils and beans all count. Supplements (like whey or collagen) can help when life gets busy.

Protein Power Rule

Aim for 1 gram of protein per pound of body weight per day.

Example: If you weigh 150 pounds, aim for ~150 grams of protein.

Don't stress if you fall short—think of it as a *goal to work toward,* not perfection. Even getting closer will help preserve muscle, control glucose, and boost satiety.

Protein Powder Isn't Just for Bodybuilders

Protein shakes, powders, or collagen can be a convenient way to hit your daily protein target. They're not a crutch—they're a tool. Especially useful for busy mornings, travel, or post-workout recovery.

Carbs Aren't the Enemy

Low-carb and keto diets have gained popularity, but here's the truth: women don't need to cut carbs completely. Carbohydrates provide energy for workouts and help regulate mood. The key is **choosing the right carbs and eating them strategically.**

- Prioritize whole-food carbs: vegetables, fruit, legumes, oats, quinoa.

- Pair carbs with protein or fat to control glucose spikes.

- Try eating carbs *later in the meal* instead of first—research shows this simple sequencing reduces glucose excursions.

For some women, reducing refined carbs or trying time-restricted eating (like a 12–14 hour overnight fast) works wonders for glucose control. For others, the Mediterranean-style diet, rich in plants, fish, and olive oil, is ideal. The point is personalization: find what stabilizes your glucose while still fueling your lifestyle.

Myth Buster: Carbs Are the Enemy

Cutting carbs completely isn't the answer.

The real key: choose quality carbs (whole fruits, veggies, legumes, oats, quinoa) and pair them with protein or fat to prevent glucose spikes. Carbs aren't evil—they just need supervision.

Meal Sequencing Hack

Eat protein + veggies **before** carbs.
Research shows this simple swap lowers glucose spikes by as much as 30–40%.

Salad and chicken before pasta > pasta first. Your body will thank you.

Fat & Fiber: The Unsung Heroes

Healthy fats (avocado, nuts, seeds, olive oil, fatty fish) slow down digestion and make meals more satisfying. Fiber—especially from vegetables and whole grains—feeds your gut microbiome and lowers post-meal glucose. Together, they act like brakes on the glucose rollercoaster.

Myth Buster: Skipping Meals Saves Calories

Skipping meals often backfires: glucose crashes → cravings → overeating later.

Balanced meals with protein + fiber keep glucose steady, hormones happy, and your willpower intact.

Case Study: Elena, 50 — "Balancing Carbs and Protein Changed Everything"

Elena had always eaten "healthy" by conventional standards: cereal for breakfast, a salad with fruit at lunch, pasta for dinner. But at 50, her weight climbed, and her doctor warned her about rising A1C levels.

After learning about glucose control, she made one change: prioritizing protein. Breakfast shifted to Greek yogurt with berries and chia seeds. Lunch became grilled chicken over greens with beans. Pasta nights stayed—but only after a plate of vegetables and lean protein first.

Within three months, Elena's energy soared, her cravings calmed, and her A1C dropped back into the normal range. She didn't eliminate carbs—she learned how to balance them.

DID YOU KNOW? Fat + Fiber = Glucose Brakes

Healthy fats + veggies slow digestion and flatten glucose spikes.

Example: Add avocado to eggs, olive oil to salads, or nuts to yogurt.

Every meal needs a brake pedal.

DID YOU KNOW? Calories Aren't the Whole Story

A 300-calorie candy bar and a 300-calorie chicken breast have radically different effects on your glucose and hormones. It's not just about "calories in, calories out"—it's about what those calories signal your body to do.

The Science of Joy

Joy might be the most underrated metabolic enhancer on the planet.

Laughter lowers cortisol. Gratitude increases dopamine and serotonin. Meaningful connection releases oxytocin — a hormone that not only softens stress but improves insulin sensitivity.

The irony? The very emotions we associate with pleasure are the ones that support fat loss, hormonal balance, and longevity. When you eat with joy — not guilt — your digestive enzymes activate more fully, your blood sugar response stabilizes, and your nervous system shifts into balance. When you move in ways that make you smile — not suffer — your consistency becomes effortless, and your body begins to trust that movement means freedom, not punishment.

Joy is chemistry in motion.

Find it in the warmth of sunlight on your morning walk, in the rhythm of your favorite song, in the laughter shared with friends, or in a quiet exhale at the end of a long day. Each moment tells your body, "You're safe. You can thrive now."

Science calls it neuroendocrine balance.
You'll feel it as joy.

"Joy is not frivolous — it's hormonal alignment disguised as happiness."

Chapter 5 Summary

Chapter Reflection: Nutrition for Hormone Balance and Glucose Control

If there's one truth this chapter revealed, it's that food is far more than fuel — it's communication. Every bite you take tells your body what to do next: store energy or burn it, repair muscle or break it down, stabilize hormones or send them into chaos.

Here, you learned that nutrition isn't about deprivation — it's about direction. When protein takes center stage, glucose stabilizes, cravings fade, and energy levels rise. Carbohydrates aren't the enemy, but unmanaged ones can send your blood sugar on a rollercoaster that leaves you tired, hungry, and inflamed. The key isn't cutting them out — it's learning how to pair them wisely and time them intentionally.

You also discovered that women's bodies respond differently to popular diet philosophies. Low-carb, Mediterranean, intermittent fasting — each can work, but not all work for you. The secret isn't in following a rulebook; it's in learning how your body feels and responds. Reinvented isn't about restriction — it's about refinement.

Elena's story brought the science home. By simply rebalancing her plate — more protein, fewer refined carbs, and better timing

— she didn't just lose belly fat; she lowered her A1C and gained steady, sustainable energy. Her shift wasn't dramatic — it was deliberate. And that made all the difference.

In the end, this chapter reminded us that nourishment is not a moral test — it's a relationship. Food is how we speak to our metabolism, soothe our hormones, and honor the vessel we live in.

When you eat with awareness and respect, your body listens — and it rewards you with balance, vitality, and strength that radiates from the inside out.

Hormone Harmony

Your hormones are not unpredictable — they are responsive. They are the rhythm your body has been dancing to all along. These reflections are a chance to tune in to that rhythm — to honor the messages your body sends and find compassion for its ebb and flow through every stage of womanhood.

Reflect + Reinvent

1. How does your energy shift through your monthly or weekly rhythm?

2. What signs tell you your body might be under stress?

3. What does "balanced" feel like for you — in energy, mood, and mindset?

4. When do you feel most in tune with your body — and when do you feel disconnected?

5. How can you honor your natural cycles instead of resisting them?

"Balance isn't found in control — it's found in conversation with your body."

"Nothing can dim the light which shines from within."

— Maya Angelou

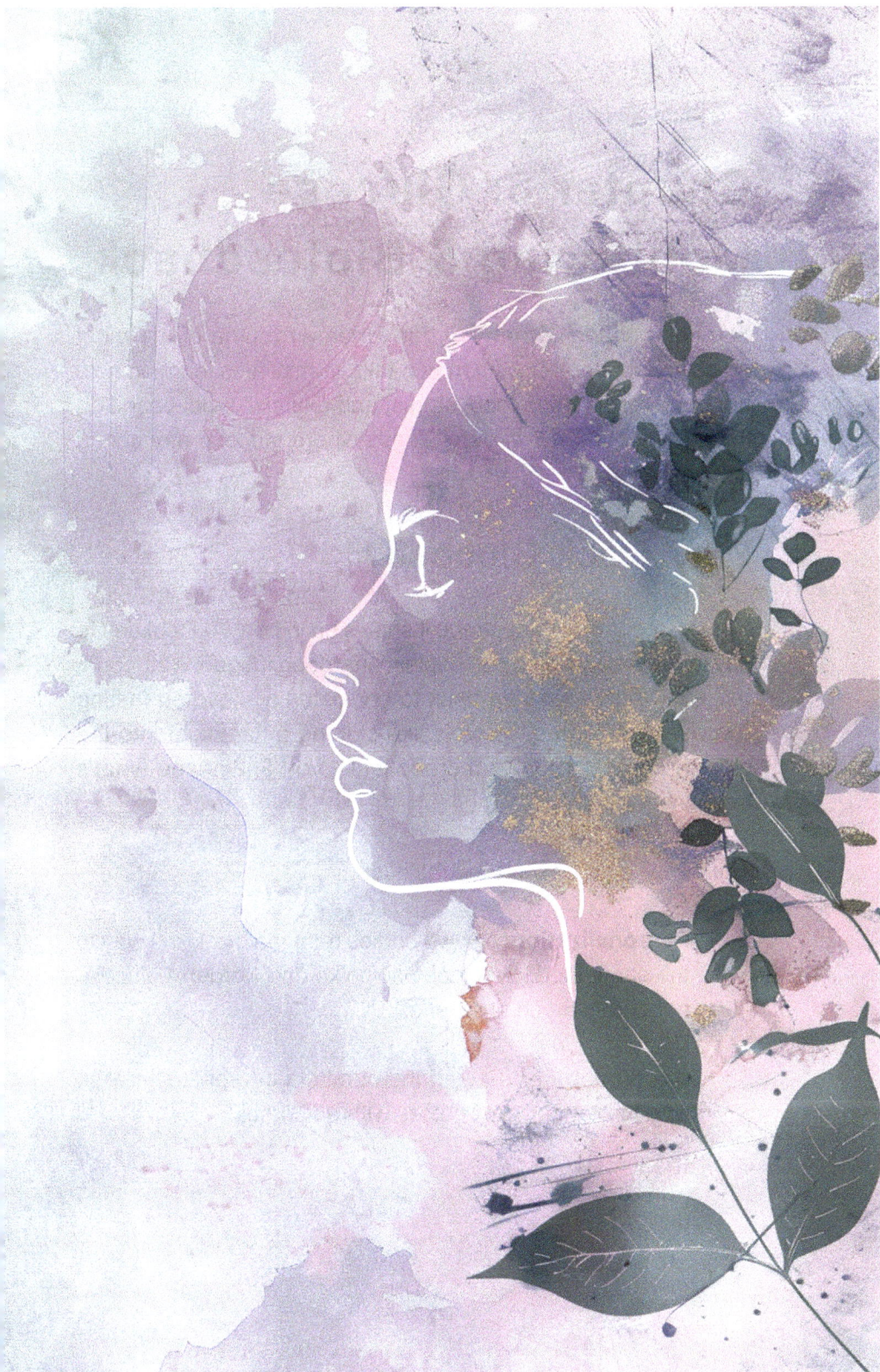

Chapter 6: Glucose Monitoring & Biofeedback

You can't change what you don't measure. One of the most empowering steps a woman can take in midlife is learning how her body responds to food, stress, and exercise—not based on theory, but on her own data. That's where glucose monitoring comes in.

Why Track Glucose?

Glucose control isn't abstract; it shows up in how you feel day to day. A post-meal crash can explain afternoon fatigue. A stubborn belly fat pattern may tie back to consistently elevated fasting glucose. Tracking glucose is like shining a flashlight into the hidden corners of your metabolism—you finally see what's happening inside.

The benefits go beyond weight loss:

- **Personalization:** No two bodies respond the same way to the same food. Oatmeal may spike one woman's glucose but barely touch another's.

- **Accountability:** Seeing the numbers in real-time makes it easier to connect choices with outcomes.

- **Motivation:** Small wins (like a lower glucose reading after a protein-rich breakfast) build momentum and confidence.

Glucose Checkpoints

When should you test?

- **Fasting (first thing in the morning):** Aim <100 mg/dL (optimal: 80–90).

- **Pre-meal:** Baseline check.

- **1–2 hours post-meal:** See how food affects you (goal: <30 mg/dL rise from baseline).

- **Bedtime:** Stable readings at night = better sleep + recovery.

How to Monitor

1. **Finger-Prick Glucometers** – Affordable and accessible. Great for spot checks (fasting, pre/post meals).

2. **Continuous Glucose Monitors (CGMs)** – Worn on the arm, they provide 24/7 glucose feedback. They're not just for diabetics—many women use them for a few weeks to identify patterns, then adjust habits accordingly.

3. **Food + Mood Journals** – Pairing subjective notes (energy, cravings, mood) with glucose readings helps connect the dots beyond the numbers.

CGM vs. Fingerstick

Finger-Prick Glucometers
- Inexpensive
- Good for spot checks
- Only a snapshot in time

Continuous Glucose Monitors (CGMs)
- 24/7 real-time data
- Reveals trends & food patterns
- Eye-opening for lifestyle effects (sleep, stress, workouts)
- Costly, may require prescription

Tip: Use a CGM for 2–4 weeks as a "metabolic audit," then switch to spot checks.

The Patterns That Matter

You don't need to obsess over every number. Focus on these trends:

- **Fasting glucose:** Aim for <100 mg/dL (optimal is 80–90).

- **Post-meal spikes:** Try to keep increases within 30 mg/dL of your baseline.

- **Recovery time:** Glucose should return to baseline within 2–3 hours after eating.

- **Steady glucose > roller coasters:** The fewer dramatic spikes and crashes, the steadier your energy and fat loss progress.

Biofeedback Pairing

Don't just track numbers—track how you feel.

- Energy level (steady or crashing?)

- Hunger (are cravings tied to spikes?)

- Mood (irritable or calm?)

- Sleep quality (restless vs. restorative)

Glucose is data. How you feel is the real feedback.

Lifestyle Habits That Lower Glucose

The science is simple but powerful:

- **Walk after eating:** Even a 10-minute walk lowers glucose.

- **Protein first:** Eating protein or fiber before carbs cuts spikes significantly.

- **Strength train:** Muscles act like glucose sponges, pulling sugar into cells without needing as much insulin.

- **Sleep & stress:** Poor sleep and high cortisol push glucose up, even with the same meals.

Lowering Glucose Habits

Small changes = big results

- **Exercise After Eating:** 10–15 min walk lowers spikes.

- **Protein first:** Eat protein/veggies before carbs.

- **Strength train:** More muscle = better glucose buffering.

- **Cinnamon:** Studies show it can reduce post-meal glucose.

- **Sleep:** 7–9 hrs/night improves insulin sensitivity.

Case Study: Rita, 47 — "Discovering Her Trigger Foods"

Rita considered herself a "healthy eater," but she always felt sluggish after lunch and couldn't shed belly fat despite daily workouts. Curious, she tried a continuous glucose monitor for two weeks.

The results surprised her: her favorite "healthy" smoothie (banana, orange juice, and yogurt) spiked her glucose higher than ice cream. Meanwhile, steak with vegetables barely caused a blip. By swapping her smoothie for eggs and adding short walks after dinner, Rita lowered her glucose numbers. Within months, her afternoon crashes disappeared, and she lost the stubborn midsection weight that had plagued her.

Her lesson—and now yours: food isn't good or bad until you see how it affects your body.

💡 The Roller Coaster Test

If your glucose is on a roller coaster, your day might feel like one too:

- 📈 **Spikes** = energy surges, cravings
- 📈 **Crashes** = fatigue, irritability, brain fog
- ✅ **Flat curves** = steady energy, better fat burning, fewer cravings

💡 Pro Tip: The Walking Sandwich

🚶 Eat → Walk → Sit.
A 10-minute walk within 30 minutes of finishing a meal significantly reduces glucose spikes.

✅ Works even after indulgences.

✅ No treadmill required—just stroll the neighborhood.

Myth: Fruit Always Spikes Glucose

❌ Not true. Whole fruit, with its fiber and water content, usually causes smaller, slower glucose rises compared to juice or dried fruit.

✅ Pair fruit with protein (apple + nut butter, berries + Greek yogurt) to make it even gentler on your system.

Myth: If My Fasting Glucose Is Normal, I Don't Need to Worry

❌ Fasting glucose is only one piece of the puzzle. You can have "normal" fasting levels but still experience big post-meal spikes.

✅ Post-meal readings and overall glucose variability are just as important for fat loss, energy, and hormone balance.

Myth: All Carbs Are Bad

❌ Carbs aren't the villain—it's the context. A bowl of white rice alone will spike glucose more than rice eaten after lean protein and veggies.

✅ It's not about cutting carbs—it's about pairing, timing, and portion.

Myth: Glucose Monitoring Is Only for Diabetics

❌ Glucose tracking is for anyone who wants to understand their metabolism. Even short-term use (2–4 weeks with a CGM) can teach you which foods and habits keep you steady.

✅ Think of it as a "metabolic audit," not a medical label.

	Myth: A Crash After a Meal Means You Burned More Calories

❌ Feeling tired or shaky after eating isn't a "good burn." It's a sign of a glucose spike followed by an insulin overshoot.

✅ Stable curves keep your body in fat-burning mode longer and reduce cravings.

Glucose Quick-Start Checklist

Step 1: Test Your Baseline

- ☑ Check your fasting glucose (goal: <100 mg/dL, optimal 80–90).

- ☑ Take a post-meal reading 1–2 hours after eating (goal: <30 mg/dL rise).

- ☑ Keep a simple log: meal + glucose + how you felt (energy, mood, cravings).

Step 2: Flatten the Curve with Food

- Prioritize protein (25–30g per meal; aim for ~1g per pound of body weight daily).

- Eat protein + veggies first, carbs last.

- Choose whole-food carbs (fruit, legumes, oats, quinoa) instead of refined ones.

- Add healthy fats + fiber to slow digestion.

Step 3: Move Your Muscles

🧍 Walk for 10–15 minutes within 30 minutes of meals.

🏋️ Strength train 2–3x per week (muscles = glucose sponges).

⚡ Add HIIT 1–2x per week (10–15 min, 2–5 all-out intervals).

Step 4: Manage Stress + Sleep

😴 Aim for 7–9 hours of sleep.

🧘 Use breathwork, meditation, or stretching to lower cortisol.

🌙 Keep a consistent bedtime routine.

Step 5: Rinse + Repeat

🔄 Test → adjust → retest. Small changes = big results.

✦ Notice how you feel as much as what the numbers say—energy, hunger, mood are part of your feedback loop.

🍋 Print this page, stick it on your fridge, or keep it in your journal. Remember: glucose isn't about perfection—it's about progress. Every spike you flatten is a step closer to steady energy, fat loss, and hormone harmony. - click here for a downloadable PDF.

Optimal Glucose Rhythm Template — this shows how a healthy, fat-burning-friendly day looks when you track readings around meals.

The Ideal Glucose Rhythm

0 hr (Pre-Meal Baseline)

- Typical range: 75 – 90 mg/dL

- You're in fat-burning mode: insulin is low, energy steady.

- If you've worked out or fasted, readings can be low-80s or upper-70s — that's perfect.

+30–60 min (Early Rise)

- Gentle rise to 100 – 115 mg/dL

- Controlled spike = your body responding normally to carbs and protein.

- A big jump (>130–140) means the meal had more quick carbs or sugar than ideal.

+90 min (Peak)

- Most people peak here.

- Optimal: 105 – 120 mg/dL

- Still fine: ≤ 140 mg/dL (as long as it's brief).

- Shorter peaks = lower insulin exposure.

+120 – 180 min (Recovery Window)

- Glucose should be back near baseline within 2 – 3 hours:

  ○ 80 – 95 mg/dL is ideal.

  ○ Within ~10 mg/dL of your pre-meal value.

- This shows insulin has cleared and fat burning can restart.

Overnight / Fasting Next Morning

- 75 – 90 mg/dL = optimal metabolic flexibility.

- If fasting glucose stays > 95 – 100 mg/dL, it can hint at cortisol stress or late-night eating.

The "Perfect Glucose Rhythm"

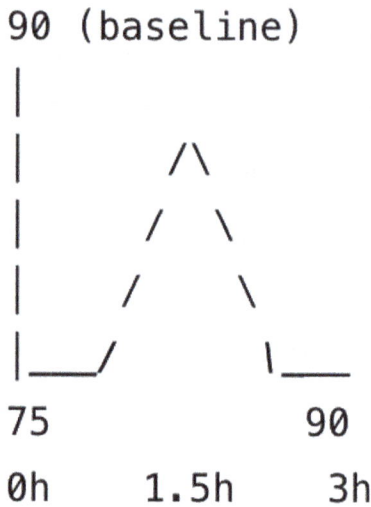

```
90 (baseline)
|
|           /\
|          /  \
|         /    \
|__/           \__
75                  90
0h        1.5h      3h
```

Smooth rise → gentle peak → steady return

❌ Sharp spike → plateau → delayed drop = excess insulin, less fat burning

How to Stay in Optimal Glucose Rhythm

- Order: veggies/fiber → protein/fat → carbs last

- Add movement: 10-15 min walk post-meal

- Hydrate: supports clearance

- Monitor: occasional checks at 0h / 1h / 2-3h tell you if your meals are in the "flat" zone

At night, Glucose stays higher longer because nighttime insulin sensitivity is lower than daytime.

Day vs. Night Glucose Curve

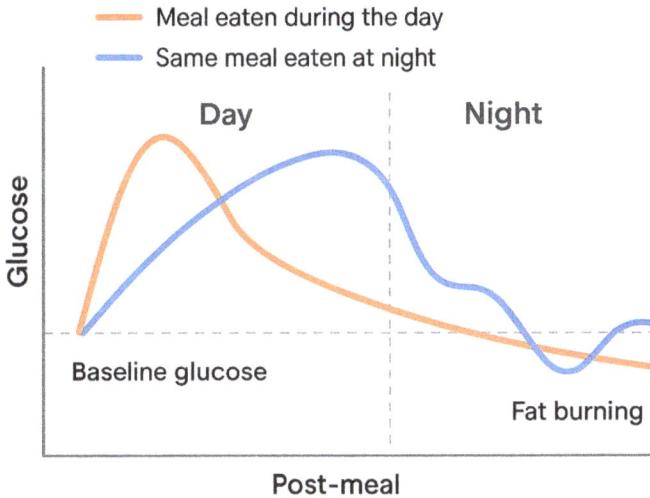

Legend:
— Meal eaten during the day
— Same meal eaten at night

Day | Night

Glucose (y-axis)

Baseline glucose

Fat burning

Post-meal (x-axis)

One of the most important and often misunderstood aspects of metabolic health. Let's break down what it means and why it matters so much for fat loss, recovery, and glucose control at night.

- "Nighttime insulin sensitivity is lower than daytime"

Your insulin sensitivity refers to how effectively your cells respond to insulin's signal to absorb glucose from the bloodstream.

- When sensitivity is high, your body needs only a little insulin to clear glucose.

- When it's low, your body has to release more insulin for the same glucose load.

At night, several biological rhythms shift that make you naturally less insulin sensitive.

1. Circadian rhythm effect

- Your metabolism follows a 24-hour rhythm controlled by your circadian clock.

- During daylight, your body expects food → muscles, liver, and fat cells are primed to handle glucose efficiently.

- After sunset, your body transitions to a repair and rest state, not a fuel-storage mode.

    o   Melatonin (the sleep hormone) rises.

    o   Insulin receptors on cells become less responsive.

    o   The pancreas itself releases less insulin.

Result:

A meal eaten at 9 pm can cause a *higher and longer-lasting glucose elevation* than the exact same meal at noon.

2. Nighttime glucose stays higher longer

Because your cells aren't as quick to absorb glucose:

- Glucose can stay elevated for 2–4 hours longer.

- Insulin remains active later into the night, which can:

  - Suppress fat burning.

  - Interfere with deep sleep stages.

  - Reduce overnight growth hormone release (needed for muscle repair).

That's why late-night eating—especially carb-heavy meals—can raise fasting glucose the next morning, even if calories were moderate.

3. Impact on fat metabolism

When insulin is high, fat oxidation (burning stored fat for fuel) shuts off.

So eating a carb-heavy meal right before bed:

- Keeps insulin up all night.

- Prevents your body from entering its natural fat-burning and cellular repair phase.

In contrast, eating protein + fat only or finishing your meal earlier allows insulin to fall — and fat burning to rise — while you sleep.

Time of Day	Insulin Sensitivity	Glucose Handling	Fat Burning
Morning/ Midday	High	Fast	Easier to burn fat post-meal
Evening / Night	Low	Slower	Suppressed until insulin falls

Chapter 6 Summary

Chapter Reflection: Glucose Monitoring & Biofeedback

This chapter was about turning awareness into empowerment — translating science into something you can feel in your own body.

You learned that glucose isn't just a number — it's a conversation your body is having with every meal, every workout, and every moment of rest. By tracking your glucose — through a continuous glucose monitor (CGM) or a simple finger prick — you begin to decode your body's language. Those "spikes" after meals, known as glucose excursions, aren't failures; they're feedback. Each one tells you something valuable about how your body responds to food, stress, and movement.

You also discovered the power of small, repeatable actions — the kind that require no diet overhaul or extreme routine. A short walk after eating. A few minutes of resistance training. Eating protein or vegetables before carbs. Each of these tiny shifts blunts glucose spikes and steadies energy, training your metabolism to work with you rather than against you.

Rita's story brought this lesson to life. When she began using a CGM, she uncovered her "trigger foods" — the hidden culprits that kept her glucose (and energy) unstable. But instead of restriction, she found freedom. By understanding her data, she could make simple swaps and smarter pairings — and watched her body respond with balance, clarity, and calm.

The deeper truth of this chapter is that tracking isn't about control; it's about connection. It's learning to listen before reacting, to understand before changing. Glucose monitoring isn't a punishment — it's a mirror that reflects your progress in real time.

And as you've seen, precision is power. When you know your body's rhythm, you can design your life around energy and strength — not exhaustion or guesswork.

Because the more you learn your numbers, the more you learn *yourself*.

"Rest and self-care are so important. When you take time to replenish your spirit, it allows you to serve others from the overflow. You cannot serve from an empty vessel."

— Eleanor Brown

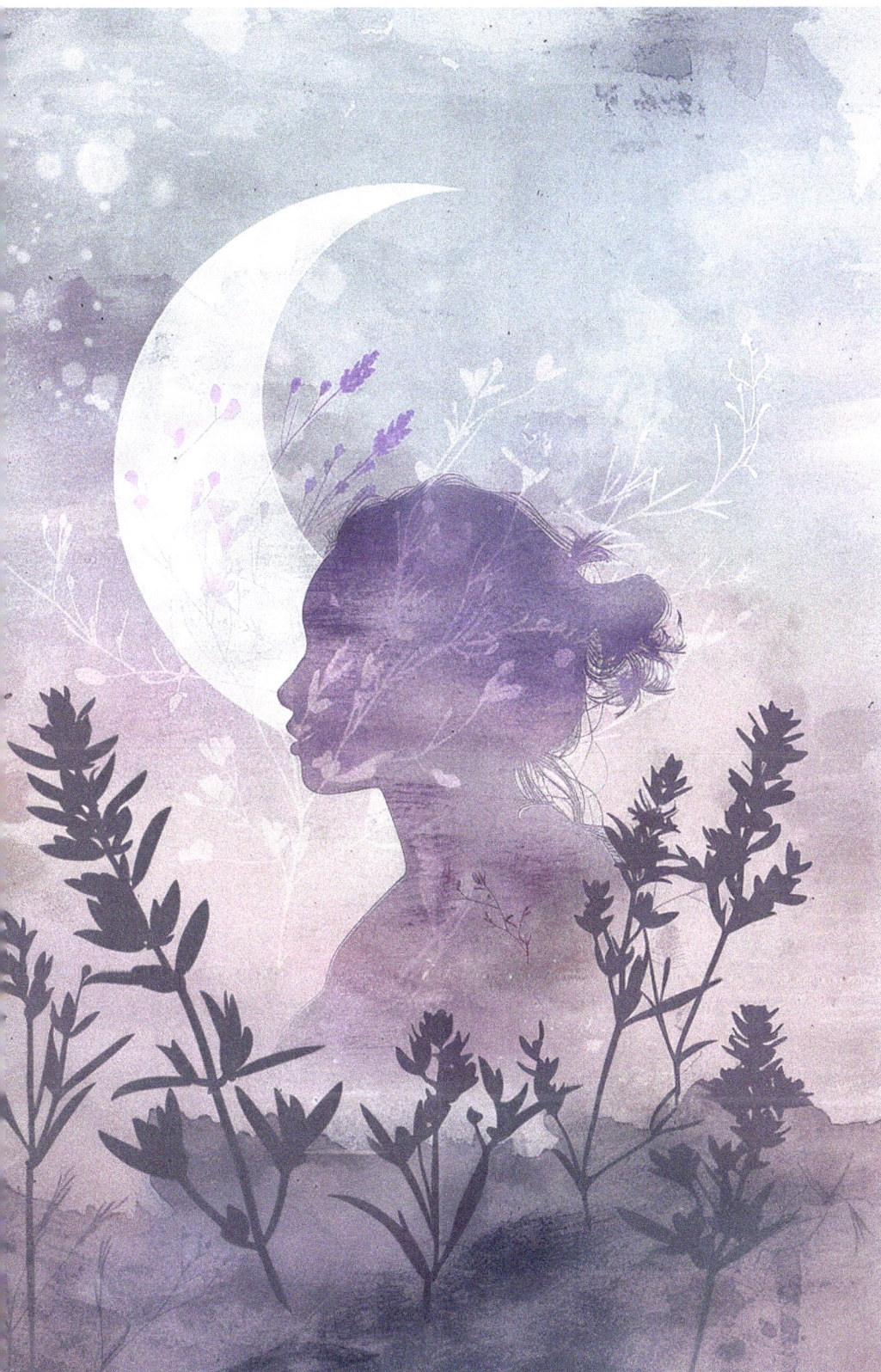

Chapter 7: Cortisol, Sleep, and Stress — The Hidden Fat Traps

Have you ever felt like you were "doing everything right"—eating well, exercising consistently—but the scale wouldn't budge? The culprit may not be your diet at all. It may be your stress.

Stress and poor sleep are silent saboteurs of weight loss, especially for women in midlife. They elevate cortisol, disrupt glucose control, and trigger cravings for quick-energy foods. The body, already adapting to lower estrogen and progesterone, becomes even more vulnerable to these hidden traps.

Cortisol: The Stress Hormone That Loves Your Belly

Cortisol isn't "bad"—it's the hormone that helps you wake up, respond to challenges, and survive emergencies. But when cortisol is chronically elevated (from stress, lack of sleep, or over-exercising), it pushes glucose levels higher, encourages insulin resistance, and signals the body to store fat—especially around the midsection.

Research shows that women under chronic stress often experience stubborn belly fat, even without overeating. That's not a failure of willpower—it's biology.

Cortisol Check-In

Signs your cortisol may be running high:

- Afternoon crashes even with good meals

- Cravings for sugar or salty snacks

- Trouble falling or staying asleep

- Belly fat that won't budge

- Feeling "tired but wired" at night

If this sounds familiar, focus on stress management before adding more workouts.

Sleep: The Overnight Reset Button

Think of sleep as the overnight glucose reset. Poor sleep increases cortisol, raises fasting glucose, and reduces insulin sensitivity the next day. It also disrupts hunger hormones: ghrelin (hunger) goes up, while leptin (satiety) goes down. The result? Stronger cravings, more snacking, and a sluggish metabolism.

Studies show that even one night of poor sleep can impair glucose regulation the next day. String together weeks or months of bad sleep, and fat loss feels nearly impossible. On the flip side, improving sleep quality is one of the fastest ways to see better glucose stability and easier fat loss.

Sleep Hygiene Quick Wins

Improve sleep (and glucose!) with these habits:

- Set a **consistent bedtime + wake time**

- Limit screens 1 hour before bed (blue light delays melatonin)

- Keep your room **cool, dark, and quiet**

- Create a "wind-down ritual" (stretching, reading, journaling)

- Avoid alcohol + heavy meals late at night

The Stress–Glucose Cycle

The challenge is circular: stress raises glucose → glucose crashes drive cravings → cravings lead to overeating → overeating worsens glucose → poor sleep makes it worse → more stress. Breaking this cycle requires more than willpower—it requires strategy.

DID YOU KNOW?	**Myth: Stress Eating Is Just Lack of Willpower**
❌	Stress eating isn't weakness—it's biology. Cortisol raises glucose, insulin responds, and your brain craves quick fuel (sugar, carbs).
✅	Learning to manage stress (breathwork, walks, sleep) lowers cravings naturally.

Practical Tools to Break the Trap

- **Stress Management:** Try breathwork (4–7–8 breathing), short walks, journaling, or meditation. Even 5 minutes can lower cortisol.

- **Exercise Smarter:** Strength training + HIIT are powerful, but too much cardio or too little recovery can spike cortisol. Balance intensity with rest.

- **Sleep Hygiene:**

  - Keep consistent bed/wake times.

  - Limit blue light before bed.

  - Create a cool, dark sleeping environment.

  - Add a wind-down routine (reading, stretching, journaling).

- **Evening Nutrition:** Avoid high-sugar foods late at night, which can spike glucose and disturb sleep cycles.

Stress Reset Mini-Tools

5-minute fixes you can do anywhere:

- **Box Breathing (4–4–4–4):** Inhale, hold, exhale, hold.

- **4–7–8 Breath:** Inhale 4, hold 7, exhale 8.

- **Micro-walk:** Step outside for 10 minutes.

- **Mind dump:** Write down tomorrow's to-do list to clear your head.

The Sleep–Glucose Loop

✦ Poor sleep → higher cortisol → higher glucose → cravings → overeating → worse sleep.

☑ Break the loop by fixing one piece (sleep or stress), and the others begin to fall in place.

Case Study: Hannah, 53 — "Stress Was My Missing Link"

Hannah was disciplined: she tracked her meals, worked out regularly, and limited treats. Yet her belly fat wouldn't budge, and she felt exhausted. A closer look revealed she was sleeping only 5–6 hours a night and working in a high-stress job.

When she began prioritizing stress reduction—daily breathing exercises, a 10-minute walk after work, and setting a strict bedtime—her transformation accelerated. Her fasting glucose dropped, her cravings diminished, and she lost the stubborn belly fat that years of dieting hadn't touched.

Her story illustrates the truth: sometimes the most powerful "workout" is turning off the lights and going to bed.

DID YOU KNOW?	**Myth: More Cardio Burns Off Stress**

❌ Long, intense cardio can actually raise cortisol if overdone.

✅ Moderate exercise + strength training + recovery help regulate stress hormones. Balance is key.

DID YOU KNOW?	**Myth: Sleep Is Optional**

❌ "I'll sleep when I'm dead" is a fast track to metabolic chaos.

✅ One bad night = impaired glucose regulation the next day. Chronic poor sleep = stubborn fat and high cortisol. Sleep is not optional—it's your nightly reset.

The Science of Rest

We've been taught that progress is made in motion — that doing more, being more, achieving more is the mark of success. But the truth is, your body does its deepest healing in stillness.

Every system you've worked so hard to optimize — glucose regulation, hormone balance, muscle repair — depends on recovery. Sleep isn't a pause; it's a performance enhancer. It's where growth hormone rises, insulin sensitivity resets, and memories and emotions organize themselves into calm clarity.

During deep sleep, your muscles rebuild from training, cortisol levels drop, and your nervous system finally exhales. Without rest, you can eat perfectly, train precisely, and still stall your results — because your body hasn't been given permission to adapt.

Rest is not a reward for hard work. It is the work.

When you honor recovery — through 7–9 hours of restorative sleep, mindful breathing, and simply stepping away from urgency — you activate the parasympathetic nervous system, the "rest-and-digest" state that signals safety to your biology. And when your body feels safe, it burns fat more efficiently, balances hormones more gracefully, and heals more completely.

Science calls it recovery.
Your body calls it peace.

"Rest is not laziness — it's where transformation takes root."

Chapter 7 Summary

Chapter Reflection: Cortisol, Sleep & Stress — The Hidden Fat Traps

If earlier chapters taught you how to fuel and move your body, this one reminded you that true transformation begins when you rest.

You learned that glucose isn't just shaped by what's on your plate — it's shaped by what's on your mind. Stress, deadlines, worries, and even overtraining can send cortisol soaring, signaling your body to hold on to fat, especially around the midsection. This isn't failure — it's biology. When the body feels under threat, it protects.

But protection isn't the same as peace. This chapter revealed that cortisol balance is the quiet key to unlocking the fat loss, energy, and mental clarity that women so often chase through effort alone. When cortisol stays elevated, glucose follows — and so do cravings, restless nights, and that sense of "doing everything right" with no results.

You discovered that rest is not laziness — it's leverage. Tools like evening wind-down rituals, strategic naps, and slow resistance training are not indulgences — they're interventions. Even something as simple as deep, steady breathing or gentle movement can shift your body from stress to safety, allowing fat metabolism and hormone repair to resume naturally.

Hannah's story brought this to life. She had spent years dieting harder and pushing longer, yet nothing worked — until she focused on her stress. When she finally prioritized sleep, recovery, and breathing as part of her training, her body responded with the fat loss and energy she'd been fighting for.

The lesson here is both simple and profound: healing doesn't happen in hustle — it happens in balance. Cortisol, sleep, and stress form the foundation of every physical transformation. When you manage them wisely, you create space for your body to do what it already knows how to do — restore itself.

So the next time you find yourself pushing harder, pause. Breathe. Remember: sometimes, the most powerful action is stillness.

The Cortisol Equation

Stress is inevitable. Burnout is optional.

Stress doesn't just live in your mind — it echoes in your body. Learning to regulate it begins with awareness. These reflections are a gentle check-in: to notice where tension hides, how it speaks, and what it might be trying to protect you from. Because peace is not found — it's practiced.

Reflect + Reinvent

1. How does stress feel in your body — physically and emotionally?

2. What situations tend to raise your cortisol most?

3. How do you typically cope with pressure, and does it serve or drain you?

4. What would it look like to practice calm before chaos — not after?

5. Where can you trade urgency for ease this week?

"The most common way people give up their power is by thinking they don't have any."

— Alice Walker

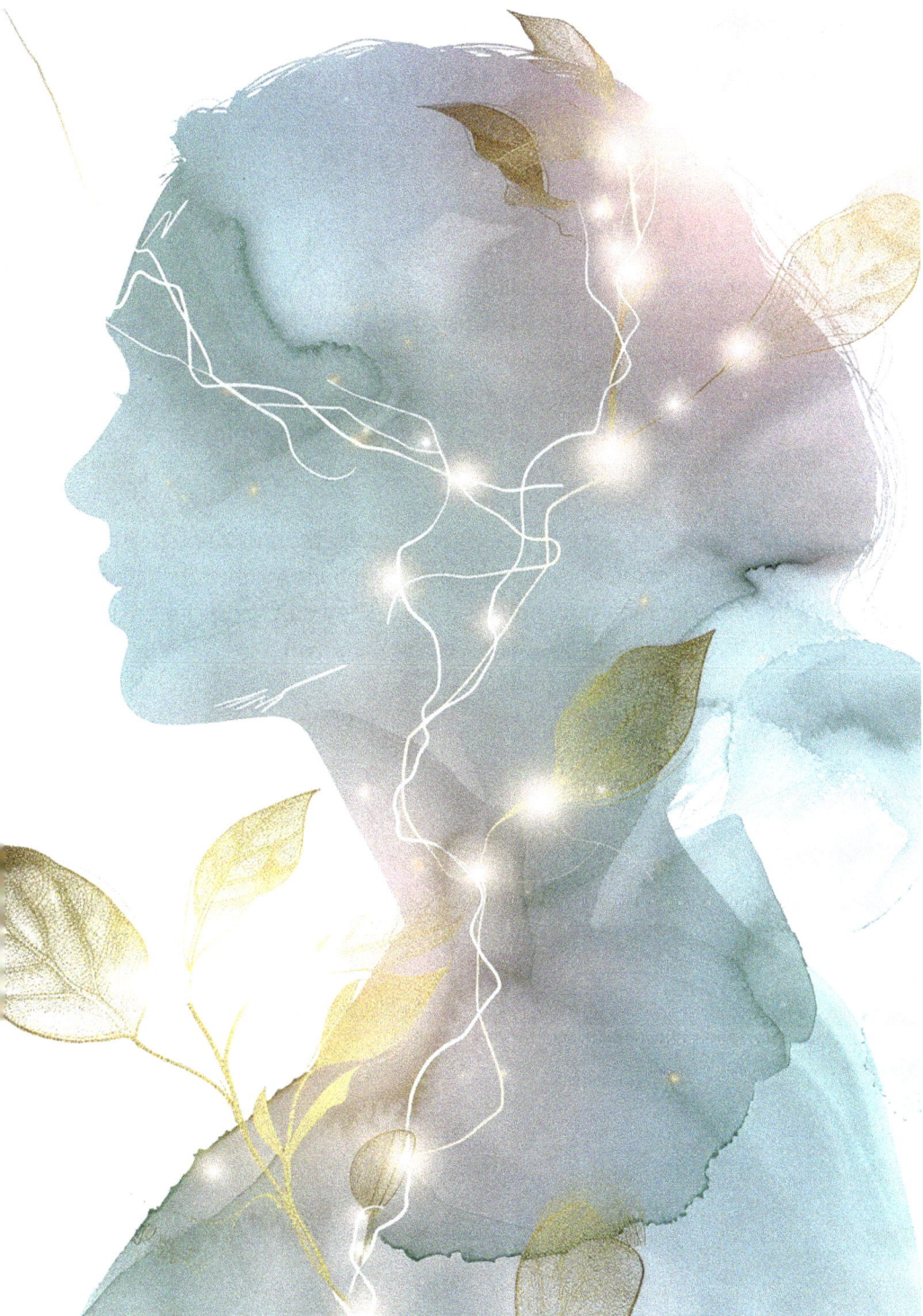

Chapter 8: Hormone Therapy & Medical Interventions

When women reach midlife, one of the first questions that often comes up is: *"Should I take hormones?"* The truth is, there's no one-size-fits-all answer. Hormone therapy, new weight-loss medications, and targeted supplements can all play a role in body transformation—but only when layered on top of a solid lifestyle foundation.

Think of it this way: if diet, exercise, stress, and sleep are the foundation of the house, medical interventions are the renovations you may or may not choose to add. They can make life easier, but they can't hold the house up on their own.

Hormone Replacement Therapy (HRT)

HRT has long been debated, but research now shows that for many women, it can be both safe and beneficial when started around the time of menopause. Benefits may include:

- Reduced hot flashes, night sweats, and sleep disturbances

- Improved mood and energy

- Better bone density and muscle maintenance

However, risks depend on type (estrogen-only vs. combined with progesterone), dosage, and individual health history. HRT is not a free pass for weight loss—it's a supportive tool that, when combined with glucose control and strength training, can make transformation easier.

Let's Talk Hormones — When "Normal" Doesn't Feel Normal

Have you ever gone to the doctor because something just didn't feel right—fatigue, mood changes, weight gain, brain fog, or trouble sleeping—only to be told that your lab work is "within normal range"?

You leave relieved that nothing serious was found, yet frustrated because you still don't feel like yourself.

This experience is incredibly common, especially for women navigating hormonal shifts. Standard lab ranges are designed to detect disease, not to measure optimal wellness. You may technically fall within what is considered "normal," while your body is quietly showing signs of imbalance.

Hormones, thyroid function, adrenal health, and nutrient levels can all influence how you feel long before traditional lab values fall outside of the expected range.

This is where a deeper, more integrative approach is needed— one that looks beyond numbers and listens to symptoms, history, and how your body is actually functioning.

You are not alone, and you are not imagining it. Feeling "not yourself" is a signal, not a weakness—and it deserves to be understood, not dismissed.

Hormone receptors are found on almost every cell in the human body.

These receptors act like tiny "locks" on the surface or inside of cells. When the correct hormone—the "key"—binds to its receptor, it sends instructions that tell the cell what to do. This is how hormones regulate essential functions such as energy, metabolism, mood, sleep, immune responses, growth, and reproduction.

Because hormone receptors exist in the brain, heart, bones, skin, muscles, and even the immune system, a hormone imbalance can affect much more than just the reproductive organs. This is why symptoms of hormone decline or deficiency—such as fatigue, anxiety, weight gain, hot flashes, or memory issues—can feel so widespread and interconnected.

In short, hormones aren't just about fertility or menopause—they are vital communicators that help every cell function properly.

Hormone Deficiency in Women — A Holistic View

Hormones quietly guide much of a woman's emotional, mental, and physical well-being. When these natural rhythms fall out of balance—through stress, aging, or lifestyle— the body begins to speak through subtle yet powerful signs.

Common Symptoms

- **Emotional changes:** Mood swings, irritability, or a sense of mental fog and disconnect.

- **Intimacy challenges:** Low libido and vaginal dryness, often causing discomfort or distance in relationships.

- **Body changes:** Unexplained weight gain, constant fatigue, and feeling "slowed down" despite rest.

- **Sleep and heat disturbances:** Difficulty sleeping, night sweats, and sudden hot flashes that disrupt peace and rest.

Listening to the Body

These symptoms are not flaws or failures—they are messages. Hormones work in harmony with the nervous system, sleep cycles, digestion, and emotions. When they shift, the whole body feels it.

Honoring these signals with nourishment, stress reduction, restful sleep, movement, and when needed, professional guidance, helps restore balance and vitality.

Symptoms of Hormone Deficiency in Women

Hormones play a vital role in regulating nearly every function in a woman's body—from mood and metabolism to sleep and reproductive health. When hormone levels decline or become imbalanced, it can lead to a range of physical, emotional, and cognitive symptoms. The following are some of the most common signs of hormone deficiency in women:

1. Mood Swings and Brain Fog

Many women experiencing hormonal imbalance report sudden shifts in mood, heightened irritability, anxiety, or feelings of depression. Along with emotional changes, some also experience "brain fog"—difficulty concentrating, forgetfulness, or mental fatigue. These symptoms are often linked to declining levels of estrogen and progesterone, which influence neurotransmitters such as serotonin and dopamine.

2. Low Libido and Vaginal Dryness

A decrease in sexual desire is one of the most commonly reported symptoms of hormone deficiency, particularly during perimenopause and menopause. Lower estrogen and testosterone levels can lead to reduced sexual interest, as well as physical discomfort during intimacy due to vaginal dryness or thinning of the vaginal tissues. These changes can affect emotional well-being and relationships if left unaddressed.

3. Weight Gain and Persistent Fatigue

Hormonal imbalance can make it difficult to maintain a healthy weight, especially around the abdomen, hips, and thighs. Slower metabolism, insulin resistance, and changes in cortisol (the stress hormone) all contribute to unwanted weight gain. In addition, chronic fatigue—feeling tired even after adequate sleep—can result from disrupted thyroid function or low estrogen levels.

4. Insomnia and Hot Flashes

Sleep disturbances are another hallmark of hormonal shifts. Women may struggle to fall asleep, wake frequently during the night, or experience poor-quality rest. Hot flashes and night sweats—sudden waves of heat, often accompanied by sweating and a pounding heartbeat—can further interrupt sleep. These symptoms are commonly associated with fluctuating estrogen levels during menopause.

Why These Symptoms Matter

While these symptoms are common, they should not be ignored or accepted as "normal" aging. Hormone deficiencies can influence cardiovascular health, bone density, cognitive function, sexual health, and overall quality of life. Recognizing the signs early allows women to seek proper evaluation, lifestyle support, and, when appropriate, medical or hormonal treatment.

Women Who May Benefit from HRT

1. Perimenopause

The years leading up to menopause can be marked by fluctuating estrogen and progesterone levels. Women may experience mood swings, irregular periods, anxiety, hot flashes, and sleep disturbances. HRT can help regulate these fluctuations and provide relief.

2. Menopause

During menopause—defined by 12 months without a menstrual cycle—hormone levels drop significantly. HRT is often used to reduce symptoms such as hot flashes, vaginal dryness, mood changes, and decreased libido.

3. Post-Menopause

After menopause, estrogen and progesterone remain low. Women may continue to experience symptoms or develop issues like bone loss, joint pain, or urogenital discomfort. HRT can be considered to support bone density, heart health, and quality of life, especially in early post-menopause.

4. Adrenal Imbalances

Chronic stress can deplete adrenal function, leading to fatigue, low energy, anxiety, sleep disturbances, and imbalanced cortisol and DHEA levels. Because adrenal hormones influence estrogen, progesterone, and testosterone production, some women with adrenal dysfunction may benefit from hormone support when lifestyle and nutritional therapies alone are not enough.

5. Thyroid Disorders

Hypothyroidism and other thyroid imbalances can mimic or worsen menopausal symptoms—such as weight gain, fatigue, hair loss, mood changes, and low body temperature. In some cases, when thyroid function affects reproductive hormone balance, carefully monitored HRT may be part of a broader treatment plan alongside thyroid support.

A Holistic Perspective

HRT is most effective when paired with a whole-person approach. This includes:

- Nourishing foods that support hormone production and liver detoxification

- Stress management to stabilize cortisol and adrenal health

- Restful sleep routines and gentle movement

- Functional lab testing and individualized medical supervision

HRT isn't about replacing what the body has lost—it's about helping the body return to harmony.

How Hormone Replacement Therapy Works

Hormone Replacement Therapy (HRT) is designed to restore balance by replacing hormones that the body no longer produces in sufficient amounts.

As women age—or when the adrenal glands, ovaries, or thyroid become imbalanced—key hormones begin to decline. This shift can lead to symptoms such as fatigue, hot flashes, mood changes, low libido, weight gain, and brain fog.

HRT works by gently reintroducing the following hormones to optimal levels:

- **Estrogen** – Supports mood, bone health, skin elasticity, and reduces hot flashes and night sweats.

- **Progesterone** – Helps regulate sleep, calms the nervous system, protects the uterine lining, and balances the effects of estrogen.

- **Testosterone** – Though present in smaller amounts in women, it is essential for energy, muscle strength, libido, and mental clarity.

- **DHEA (Dehydroepiandrosterone)** – A precursor hormone produced by the adrenal glands; it helps the body convert into estrogen and testosterone, supports mood, immunity, and overall vitality.

- **Thyroid (Desiccated Thyroid Hormone)** – A natural form of thyroid replacement containing both T3 and T4 hormones. It supports metabolism, energy production, body temperature regulation, mental clarity, and healthy weight maintenance. Low thyroid function often mimics or worsens menopausal symptoms, making thyroid support an important part of hormonal therapy for some individuals.

By replacing what the body is lacking, HRT aims to bring the endocrine system back into harmony—easing symptoms and supporting physical, emotional, and cognitive well-being.

Historical Concerns: The WHI Study (2002)

In 2002, the Women's Health Initiative (WHI) released a landmark study that dramatically changed the perception of hormone replacement therapy (HRT).

Initial Findings

- Women taking **estrogen plus synthetic progestin (EPT)** showed an increased risk of invasive breast cancer.

- Cancers found in the EPT group tended to be more advanced.

- Women taking **estrogen alone (ET)** did **not** have an increased risk—and some data suggested a slight reduction in breast cancer risk.

Impact

The study sparked widespread fear and confusion. Many women and healthcare providers abruptly stopped HRT, leading to a significant decline in its use worldwide.

Re-Evaluating the WHI: What We Know Now

In the years following the WHI study, researchers took a closer look at the original data. They found that some of the early conclusions were misunderstood or overstated, leading to unnecessary fear.

Updated Understanding

- The increased breast cancer risk was mainly associated with **synthetic progestin** (used in EPT), not estrogen alone.

- Women who had a hysterectomy and took **estrogen-only therapy (ET)** actually showed a **reduced risk of breast cancer and lower overall mortality.**

- Age matters: Women who began HRT **before age 60 or within 10 years of menopause** experienced the **most benefits and lowest risks.**

- The study participants were, on average, **63 years old,** many years post-menopause, which does not reflect the typical age when HRT is started.

Modern Perspective

Today, many experts agree that HRT is **safe and effective for healthy women in early menopause** when personalized and properly monitored. Newer, **bioidentical hormones and transdermal delivery methods** (like patches and creams) are considered safer options for many women.

From Fear to Balance

The WHI study brought awareness—but also confusion. Now, with a more nuanced understanding, HRT is no longer seen through a lens of fear but as a valuable therapy when used appropriately.

Benefits of Hormone Therapy for General Health

Hormone therapy not only relieves menopausal symptoms—it can also support whole-body health when carefully prescribed. Key benefits include:

- **Energy & Sleep** – Balanced cortisol and melatonin help improve daily energy, stress response, and sleep quality.

- **Mood & Clarity** – Supports neurotransmitters, reducing mood swings, anxiety, and brain fog.

- **Heart Health** – Estrogen helps protect blood vessels and supports healthy cholesterol levels.

- **Bone Strength** – Prevents bone loss and lowers the risk of osteoporosis.

- **Metabolism** – Improves insulin sensitivity, supports healthy fat distribution, and aids weight management.

- **Sexual Health & Libido** – Increases libido, improves sexual comfort and function, and enhances body confidence.

Reference: Farr, Kenneth, MD. Hormone Health and Replacement Therapy. Slide presentation, 2025

DID YOU KNOW	**Myth: HRT Will Make You Gain Weight**

❌ Not true. Research shows HRT does not directly cause weight gain.

✅ In fact, it may help reduce belly fat, preserve muscle, and improve sleep—making it easier to manage weight when combined with lifestyle changes.

GLP-1 Medications (Ozempic, Wegovy, etc.)

The buzz around GLP-1 receptor agonists is real, and for good reason. These medications mimic the hormone GLP-1, which:

- Slows gastric emptying (keeps you fuller longer)

- Reduces appetite and cravings

- Improves glucose control

- Promotes significant weight loss in many women

But here's the catch: studies show that without resistance training and protein, women on GLP-1 drugs can lose a significant amount of muscle along with fat. That makes strength training and protein intake non-negotiable for anyone considering this path.

Myth: GLP-1s Work Without Exercise

❌ Not True. GLP-1 medications (Ozempic, Wegovy, etc.) are powerful for appetite and glucose control, but they don't discriminate between fat and muscle.

✅ Without resistance training and protein, up to **30–40% of weight lost** can come from lean mass. Exercise + protein = muscle protection.

Supplements With Evidence

Not all supplements are snake oil.
Some have well-documented benefits for glucose, hormone balance, and overall metabolic health — especially when paired with sound nutrition, movement, and rest.

Berberine:
Shown to lower blood glucose and improve insulin sensitivity — often called "nature's metformin."

Creatine:
Supports lean muscle strength, recovery, and cellular energy — particularly valuable for women over 40 to maintain muscle mass and brain health.

Omega-3s:
Anti-inflammatory fats that support heart, brain, and hormone health while reducing insulin resistance.

Vitamin D + K2:
Essential duo for bone strength, immune function, and metabolic balance.

Magnesium:
Promotes relaxation, improves sleep quality, eases muscle tension, and supports glucose regulation.

L-Theanine:
A calming amino acid naturally found in green tea. Helps reduce stress, improve focus, and enhance sleep quality by increasing alpha-wave activity in the brain — leading to a calmer mind and steadier glucose response overnight.

> *Supplements should support, not replace,*
> *lifestyle habits. Think of them as quiet allies*
> *that amplify the effects of balanced nutrition,*
> *restorative sleep, and mindful movement.*

Supplements aren't magic—but they can fill gaps and give your metabolism an edge.

Myth: Supplements Can Replace Lifestyle

✅ No supplement can outwork poor nutrition, lack of sleep, or stress.

❌ Supplements supplement—they fill gaps, but the foundation is still food, movement, and recovery.

Top 6 Evidence-Based Supplements for Women in Midlife

These aren't magic pills — but they are grounded in science and proven to support women's health, strength, and balance.

Creatine — Preserves muscle, boosts strength, and supports brain health.

Berberine — Improves insulin sensitivity and helps regulate blood glucose.

Vitamin D + K2 — Protects bones, supports hormones, and enhances metabolic health.

Omega-3s — Reduces inflammation while nourishing heart, brain, and mood.

Magnesium — Calms the nervous system, improves sleep, and supports glucose stability.

L-Theanine — Promotes relaxation, reduces stress, and enhances deep, restorative sleep.

Always consult your healthcare provider before starting new supplements — especially if you're taking medication or managing a chronic condition.

When to Consider Medical Support

- Severe menopausal symptoms impacting quality of life

- Persistent glucose issues or prediabetes despite lifestyle changes

- Bone density loss not improving with training/nutrition alone

- Weight gain resistant to diet and exercise, accompanied by metabolic markers (insulin resistance, high A1C, elevated cortisol)

Medical options should never be a first line—but they can be a *supportive bridge* when combined with the foundational strategies in this book.

When to Talk to Your Doctor About HRT

If you're experiencing:

- *Severe hot flashes or night sweats*

- *Sleep disruption*

- *Mood swings or depression*

- *Rapid bone density loss*

- *Persistent weight gain despite consistent lifestyle changes*

HRT works best when started around menopause, not decades later.

Case Study: Deborah, 62 — "Both/ And, Not Either/Or"

Deborah had tried everything—clean eating, strength training, walking, sleep hygiene—but her hot flashes, belly fat, and bone density scans told a different story. With her doctor, she chose to start bioidentical HRT. Within months, her symptoms improved, she recovered faster from workouts, and she felt like herself again.

But Deborah didn't stop there—she doubled down on strength training, dialed in her protein, and added creatine. The result? She lost fat, gained muscle, and improved her bone density. Deborah's story proves the point: medical interventions are most powerful when they support lifestyle, not replace it.

Pro Tip: The Both/And Approach

Think of HRT, GLP-1s, or supplements as a "support crew." They make the journey smoother—but they can't drive the car. Lifestyle is always in the driver's seat.

Chapter 8 Summary

Chapter Reflection: Hormone Therapy & Medical Interventions

This chapter reminded us that knowledge is power — and that power is amplified when it's paired with discernment.

You learned that there's no single "fix" for midlife changes, and that's a good thing. True health isn't found in one prescription, one supplement, or one path — it's built layer by layer, through informed decisions and aligned actions.

We explored how modern medicine can serve as a powerful ally. Hormone Replacement Therapy (HRT) and bioidentical options can ease symptoms and improve quality of life when used wisely. GLP-1 receptor agonists, like Ozempic or Wegovy, demonstrate just how profoundly glucose regulation can influence appetite and body composition. But the real message was clear: these tools work best with your foundation — not instead of it.

Deborah's story showed what this balance looks like in real life. By combining bioidentical HRT with strength training and mindful nutrition, she didn't just change her body; she changed her experience of aging. She found her energy again, her confidence, and her calm.

You also discovered the evidence-backed support of nutraceuticals — berberine, magnesium, omega-3s, vitamin D and K2, and creatine — gentle but powerful allies that enhance glucose control, muscle preservation, and hormone balance. They are not quick fixes, but quiet reinforcements for a body in transformation.

The deeper truth is that medicine should never silence your body's wisdom — it should amplify it. The goal isn't dependence; it's partnership. When medical tools are used intentionally, they can help restore balance faster, giving your lifestyle habits the space to take root.

In the end, this chapter invited you to see the full spectrum of options — from the natural to the clinical — and to stand in the center of it with clarity and confidence.

Because you don't have to choose between science and self-trust. You can have both.

"The most courageous act is still to think for yourself. Aloud."

— Coco Chanel

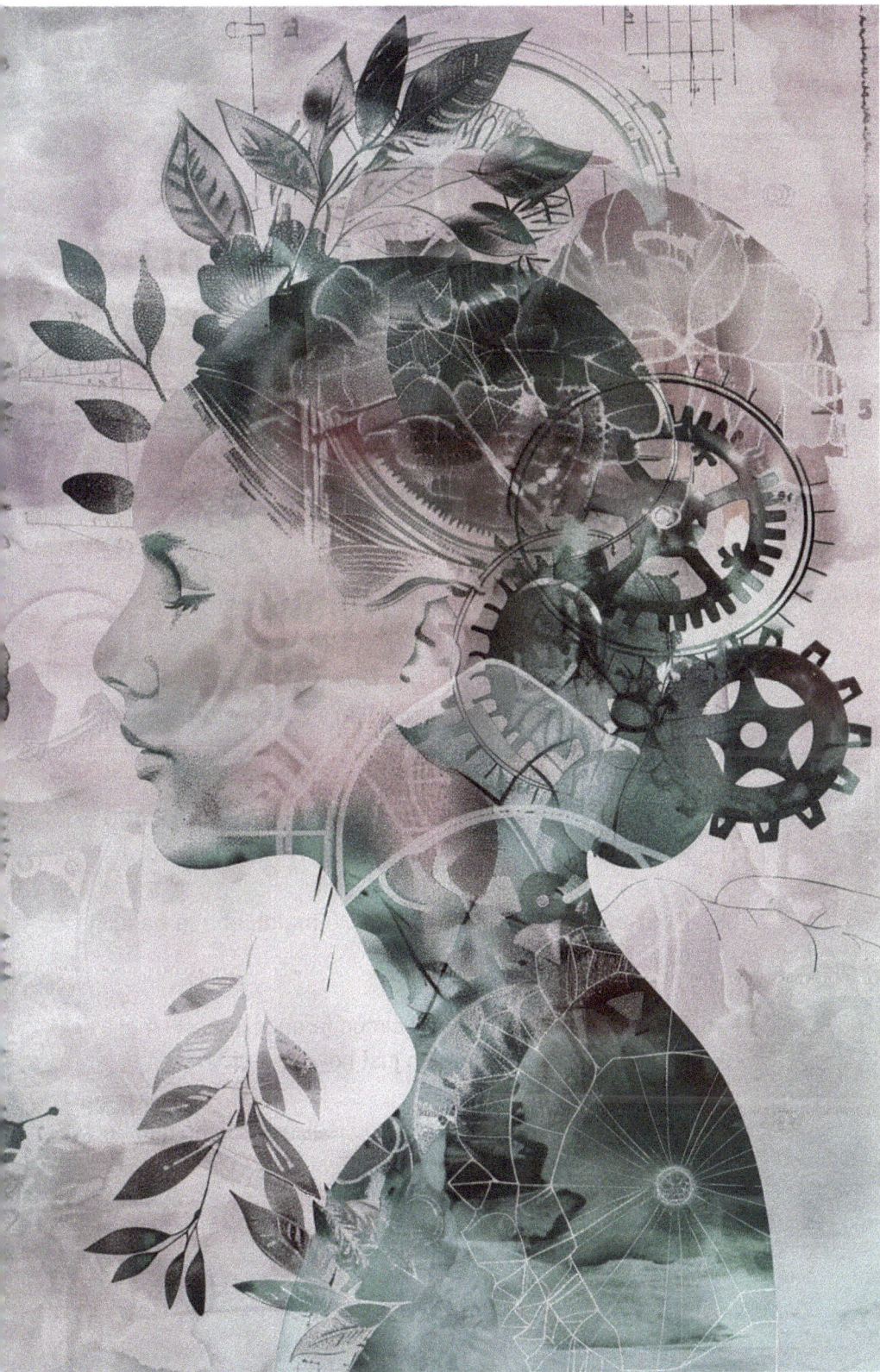

Chapter 9: Designing Your Glucose Control Blueprint

By now, you understand the science: how glucose interacts with hormones, why muscle is your metabolic currency, and how sleep, stress, and nutrition all fit together. You've seen the case studies of women just like you—each with her own challenges and solutions. Now it's time to design your **Blueprint:** a simple, customized plan that works with *your* body, your lifestyle, and *your* goals.

Step 1: Know Your Numbers

Get a glucose monitor. Find them online at Amazon or at your local pharmacy. They range from $20 - $30. Before you start tweaking, you need a baseline.

- **Fasting glucose:** Ideally 80–90 mg/dL, but <100 is acceptable.

- **Post-meal glucose:** Aim for <30 mg/dL above baseline at 1–2 hours.

- **Body composition:** Waist circumference, muscle mass (if you have access), or even just how your clothes fit.

- **Energy & mood:** Track how you feel, not just the numbers.

These are your starting "data points." No judgment, just information.

Step 2: Set Your Priorities

Not everything needs to change at once. Choose one or two areas to start, based on what matters most right now:

- Struggling with cravings? → Focus on meal sequencing & protein.

- Belly fat won't budge? → Add resistance training 2–3x/week.

- Feeling exhausted? → Improve sleep hygiene.

- High stress? → Add 5–10 min of daily stress resets (breathing, walking).

Pick the area that feels both *doable* and *impactful*. Master it, then layer on the next.

Step 3: Build Your Weekly Routine

Think of your Blueprint as a rhythm, not a rigid plan. Here's a starting point:

- **Nutrition:**
  - 25–30g protein per meal (goal: ~1g protein per pound of body weight daily).
  - Protein/veggies first, carbs last.
  - Healthy fats + fiber at every meal.

- **Exercise:**
  - 2–3 resistance training sessions per week (weights or calisthenics).
  - Move after Meals (10 - 15 min of walking, cycling, dancing).
  - 1–2 HIIT sessions (10–15 minutes, 2–5 intervals).

- **Recovery:**
  - 7–9 hrs sleep.
  - 1–2 stress resets daily.
  - One full rest day per week.

Step 4: Track, Adjust, Repeat

This isn't a one-and-done plan—it's a living blueprint.

- Test → Adjust → Retest.

- Notice not just weight changes, but energy, cravings, mood, sleep, and strength.

- Expect plateaus—they're just signals to tweak protein, training, or recovery.

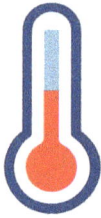

Finger–Stick Glucose Mastery Guide

🕐 Optimal test timings

😊 First thing in morning

☕ 1 hour after eating

🍴 2 hours after eating

Glucose levels

fasting	70–100 mg/dL
pre meal	80–100 mg/dL
post meal	<140 mg/dL

↗ Understanding rises and drops

↘ Minimal rise, steady range
Fat-burning metabolism

↑ Quick spike, slow recovery
Carb-reliant metabolism

↓ Drop 50+ mg/dL from peak

Myth: You Need a "Perfect Plan" Before You Start

✅ Not True. Waiting for the perfect time or program keeps you stuck.

❌ Start with one step (like walking after dinner). Build layer by layer. The perfect plan is the one you actually do.

Case Study: Paula, 58 — "My Personalized Blueprint"

Paula had tried generic meal plans and workout challenges but always fell off track. When she built her own glucose control blueprint, everything clicked. She started with protein and walking after dinner, then layered in strength training twice a week. A few months later, she added HIIT.

Instead of overhauling her entire life, Paula made small, steady changes. Her fasting glucose dropped, her waist shrank by 3 inches, and—most importantly—she felt in control for the first time in years. Two years later, she's still living by her blueprint, adjusting as her life evolves.

Build-Your-Blueprint Worksheet

Use this template to sketch your personal plan:

My Baselines

- Fasting glucose: _____

- Post-meal glucose (avg): _____

- Waist measurement: _____

- Energy/mood (scale 1–10): _____

My Top 2 Priorities

1. _____

2. _____

My Weekly Rhythm

- Strength Training: _____ days

- Cardio/Walking: _____ days

- HIIT: _____ days

- Sleep Goal: _____ hours

- Daily Stress Reset: _____ minutes

Check-In Date (2–4 weeks from now): _____

Sample Weekly Schedule

Here's what a glucose-friendly week can look like:

Mon: Strength Training (lower body)
Tue: HIIT (10–15 min)
Wed: Strength Training (upper body)
Thu: HIIT (10–15 min)
Fri: Strength Training (full body)
Sat: Walk, Fun Cardio (hike, bike, dance, pickleball)
Sun: Rest + Mobility/Stretching

Adjust based on energy, lifestyle, and goals. Consistency beats perfection.

The Longevity Add-Ons: Mobility, Flexibility & Flow

As women move through different stages of life, maintaining mobility and flexibility becomes just as essential as building strength. Incorporating **Pilates** and **yoga** into your weekly rhythm supports graceful movement, balance, and breath control — all key to a long, healthy healthspan.

- **Pilates** enhances *core stability, posture, and joint mobility,* helping your body move efficiently and age gracefully.

- **Yoga** supports *flexibility, mindfulness, and deep breath work,* reducing cortisol (your stress hormone) and improving recovery between workouts.

Once your **Glucose Blueprint** schedule feels natural, layer in these restorative practices 1–2 times per week. Think of them as your *longevity rituals* — the secret to staying strong, supple, and centered for decades to come.

Plateau Fixers

If fat loss stalls or energy dips, ask:

- Am I hitting my protein goal (1g per lb body weight)?

- Have I increased weights/reps in strength training?

- Am I truly sleeping 7–9 hrs?

- Is stress sneaking back in?

- Am I logging glucose consistently?

Often the plateau isn't failure—it's feedback.

Pro Tip: Focus on "Keystone Habits"

Some habits create ripple effects:

- Prioritizing protein → fewer cravings, steadier glucose.

- Lifting weights → better sleep, stronger bones.

- Sleeping well → lower cortisol, improved willpower.

Choose 1–2 keystone habits to anchor your blueprint.

Chapter 9 Summary

Chapter Reflection: Designing Your Glucose Control Blueprint

This chapter marked a turning point — the moment when theory became practice, and knowledge became empowerment.

Up until now, you've learned *why* glucose control matters, *how* hormones shape your metabolism, and *what* lifestyle tools make a difference. But this is where everything comes together — where you begin to design your own blueprint, one that reflects your unique body, your rhythms, and your goals.

You discovered that transformation doesn't come from doing everything at once — it comes from layering change with intention. One new habit at a time. One meal, one workout, one night of better sleep. Consistency — not perfection — creates stability, and stability creates results.

Tracking became your mirror in this process. Rather than relying solely on the scale, you learned to look at body composition, waist circumference, glucose trends, and strength progression. These data points don't judge you — they guide you. A plateau isn't proof of failure; it's an invitation to recalibrate, to listen more closely, and to refine your strategy.

Paula's story illustrated the power of sustainability. At 58, she built her own glucose-control lifestyle — not a temporary plan, but a living, breathing rhythm that carried her through two full years of strength, balance, and confidence. She didn't chase results — she lived them.

The truth is, your blueprint won't look like anyone else's — and that's exactly how it should be. This isn't about comparison; it's about coherence. The more aligned your choices are with your body's feedback, the easier everything becomes.

As you complete this chapter, know this: you now hold the map. Every principle you've learned — from glucose stability to muscle growth, from recovery to mindset — is a piece of your own design.

You're not following a plan anymore.
You're building one.

The Reinvented Blueprint

By now, you've gathered knowledge, habits, and data — but reflection turns all of that into wisdom. These prompts help you anchor what you've learned into your daily rhythm. Think of this as your calibration point — the pause before momentum, where understanding becomes embodiment.

The framework is simple — but transformation happens in consistency.

Reflect + Reinvent

1. What small habit has made the biggest difference in your energy so far?

2. What new data about your body surprised you the most?

3. How will you measure success beyond the scale?

4. What does consistency look like when life gets busy or stressful?

5. How will you celebrate small victories on this journey?

.

"I am not afraid of storms, for I am learning how to sail my ship."

— Louisa May Alcott

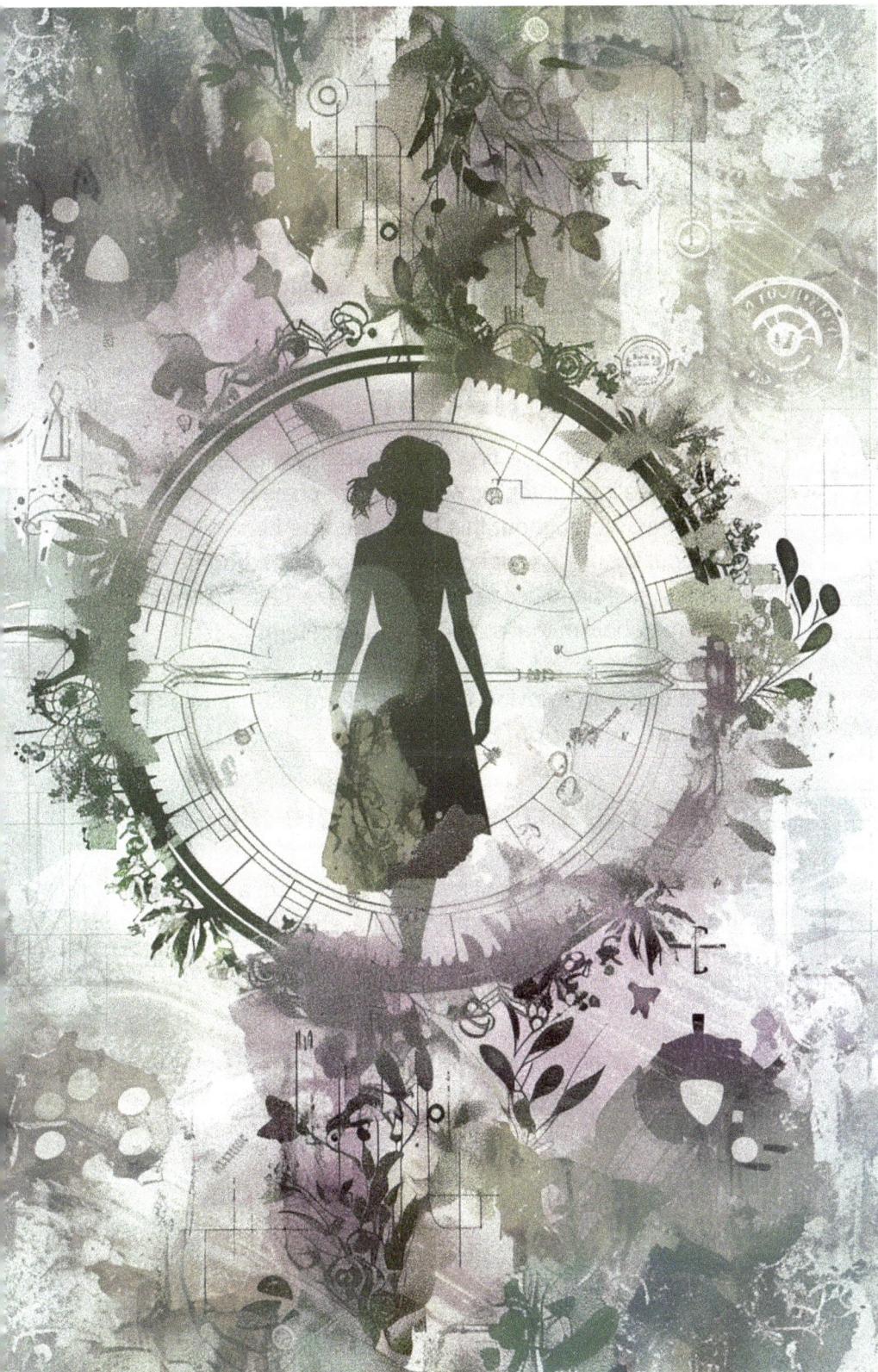

Chapter 10: Long-Term Success — From Weight Loss to Body Transformation

For many women, the first goal is weight loss—fitting into old clothes, feeling lighter, or watching the scale go down. But as you've seen throughout this book, the true transformation isn't just about shrinking your body. It's about **rebuilding it**—stronger muscles, steadier glucose, healthier bones, balanced hormones, and a metabolism that supports you long term.

This is the pivot: moving from short-term fat loss into **lifelong body transformation.**

From Fat Loss to Muscle Mastery

In the early stages, weight loss may come from a combination of fat and muscle. But over time, the goal shifts: *preserve and build lean tissue while trimming fat.* That's where strength training, protein, and glucose control become your forever tools.

Studies show that women who maintain strength training into their 50s, 60s, and beyond have better balance, higher metabolism, and lower risk of falls and fractures. Muscle isn't vanity—it's your insurance policy for independence and vitality.

Longevity Benefits Beyond the Mirror

By mastering glucose and muscle, you're not just improving your waistline—you're protecting your future.

- **Bone health:** Strength training + protein + Vitamin D = stronger bones, reduced osteoporosis risk.

- **Heart health:** Lower glucose variability = lower cardiovascular risk.

- **Brain health:** Stable glucose supports cognitive performance and reduces dementia risk.

- **Energy & mood:** Better sleep, less stress, and steady energy improve your daily life.

This isn't just about adding years to your life—it's about adding *life to your years.*

Embracing Adaptation

Here's the truth: your needs will change. What works at 45 or 50 may not be the same at 65. The magic of your Glucose Control Blueprint is that it adapts. Plateaus, setbacks, even major life shifts (like retirement, injury, or caregiving) don't derail you—they just invite you to tweak your plan.

Think of your body like an ongoing project: you don't finish it once and for all. You maintain, strengthen, and refine it, layer by layer.

Case Study: Maya, 65 — "Strong Into Retirement"

Maya thought menopause meant slowing down. But at 65, after committing to her blueprint for over a decade, she's stronger than she was at 40. Her doctor reduced her medications, she hikes with her grandkids, and she's proud of the muscle definition she built through simple, consistent training.

Maya's secret? She stopped chasing diets and started building a lifestyle. She still enjoys occasional wine with friends and family dinners, but she anchors her days with protein, movement, and sleep. Her blueprint isn't rigid—it's sustainable.

Her story shows the ultimate goal: not just losing weight, but creating a body and lifestyle that carries you powerfully into your next decades.

Your Next Chapter

This book has given you the science, the strategies, and the stories. Now, the blueprint is in your hands. As you continue, remember:

- Glucose is your lever.

- Muscle is your currency.

- Sleep and stress are your silent allies.

- Hormones and medical support are optional tools, not magic bullets.

Transformation is not about perfection. It's about progression, personalization, and consistency. The more you practice, the more effortless it becomes.

You're not just managing menopause. You're mastering your metabolism—and building a stronger, more resilient body for the next chapter of your life.

Chapter 10 Summary

Chapter Reflection: Long-Term Success — From Weight Loss to Body Transformation

This chapter brought everything full circle — from the science of glucose and muscle to the art of living well for decades to come.

You've learned that weight loss is only the beginning. The real goal — the lasting one — is transformation: a body that feels strong, a mind that feels clear, and a life that feels deeply aligned with your energy and purpose. This is the shift from "losing" to building — from counting calories to cultivating vitality.

You now understand that the habits you've practiced — strength training, balanced nutrition, glucose control, restorative sleep — do far more than shape your body. They protect your bones from osteoporosis, your muscles from decline, your brain from fog, and your heart from disease. Every rep, every meal, every mindful breath is a quiet investment in your future self.

Maya's story reminded us that it's never too late to start — and never too early to sustain. At 65, she carried her strength into retirement not by chasing youth, but by embracing her evolution. Her transformation wasn't about vanity; it was about vitality — living fully, traveling freely, and feeling at home in her body again. This chapter asked you to redefine what success looks like. Not a goal weight. Not a number. But a way of being — grounded, confident, and strong. It's about aging differently: with curiosity, with grace, and with intention.

You've built the habits that change metabolism. Now you're building the mindset that changes everything.

Because health isn't something you achieve — it's something you *live*.
And the longer you practice, the stronger, steadier, and more radiant you become.

This isn't the end of your journey.
It's the beginning of your *Reinvention*.

The Reinvention Mindset

You've gathered data, habits, and awareness. Now it's time to embody it — to live as the woman who knows her worth is not in what she loses, but in what she gains.

Reflect + Reinvent

1. What parts of yourself have you rediscovered through this process?

2. How has your definition of health evolved?

3. What does "living reinvented" look like day to day?

4. How will you protect your peace and progress in the months ahead?

5. Write a letter to your future self, one year from now, thanking her for staying committed to your reinvention.

"You are the evidence that healing is possible — and it looks good on you."

"I am deliberate and afraid of nothing."

— Audre Lorde

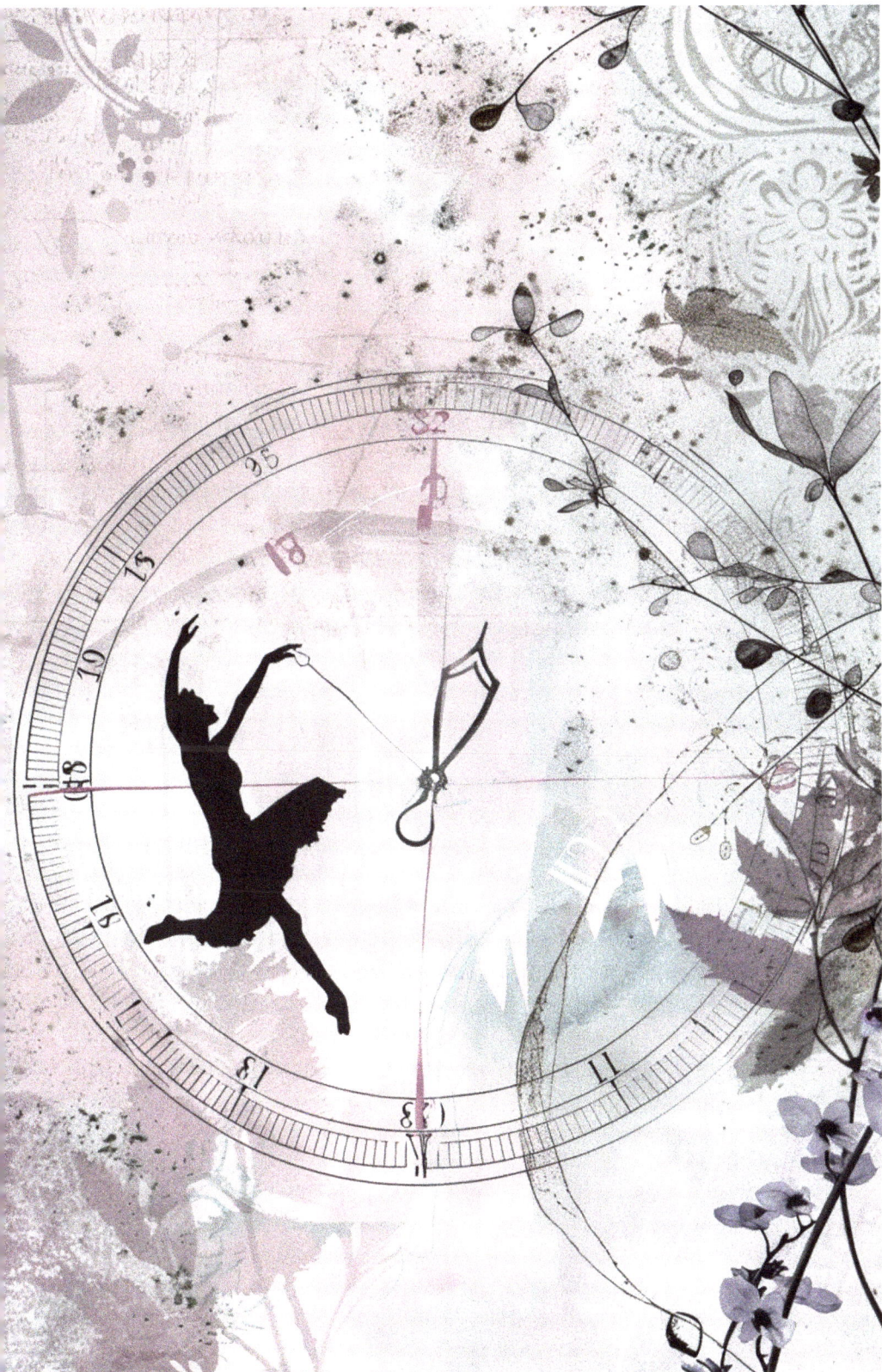

Chapter 11:
Your Next Chapter Begins Here

If you've made it this far, take a moment to celebrate. You've invested in understanding your body at a stage of life when so many women feel overlooked, dismissed, or confused. You've learned the truth: that transformation in midlife and beyond isn't just possible—it's powerful.

You now know the levers that matter most: glucose, muscle, sleep, stress, and (if needed) medical support. You've seen how women like Maria, Tanya, Janet, and Maya reclaimed their strength and energy, not through fads or extremes, but through steady, science-backed changes. And you've designed (or begun designing) your own **Glucose Control Blueprint**—a framework that adapts to *you*.

Here's our challenge to you: don't let this knowledge sit on the page. Put it into practice. Pick one thing—add protein at breakfast, walk after dinner, lift weights twice this week, go to bed 30 minutes earlier—and do it. Small, repeated actions transform your body, your energy, and your future.

This isn't the end of the book—it's the beginning of your next chapter.

What's Next: From Learning to Living

To make this blueprint come alive, the next section of this book gives you the practical tools to put everything into action:

- **Summary of Key Studies** — A curated list of women-focused research so you can see the science behind the strategies.

- **Meal Templates & Glucose-Friendly Recipes** — Easy, adaptable meals that keep your glucose steady while fueling your workouts and daily life.

- **Sample Resistance Training Programs** — Age- and level-specific workouts to help you build muscle, preserve bone, and improve strength whether you're 40, 50, 60, or beyond.

- **Tools and Tracking Worksheets** — Printable tools to log your glucose, hormones, sleep, and training progress, so you can see your blueprint evolve over time.

Your Call to Action

Transformation isn't about waiting for the perfect Monday, the right program, or the stars to align. It starts now—with the knowledge in your hands and the choice to act.

You don't have to do everything. Just start with something.

Because every stable glucose reading, every protein-rich meal, every night of deep sleep, every rep of strength training—these are deposits into your future.

And your future is strong, resilient, and unstoppable.

This is your blueprint. This is your time. Let's begin.

Resources, Studies & Reflection

The Science of Self-Tracking — Learning Your Body's Language

We've covered the framework, the science, and the stories — but this section is where the transformation becomes personal.

Because knowledge alone doesn't change your body — *awareness* does.

Self-tracking is not about perfection, guilt, or obsession. It's about building a gentle partnership with your own biology. Think of it as a dialogue: you ask your body a question (through action), and it answers (through feedback). Over time, these answers form a language — a map — that leads you toward balance, vitality, and freedom.

The key is curiosity, not criticism. Tracking your glucose, workouts, recovery, and nutrition gives you information — not identity. Numbers don't define you; they guide you. This is data wlth compassion — a way to replace frustration with insight.

When you learn to interpret what your body is saying, you stop guessing. You stop fearing the plateau, the craving, the energy dip. You stop trying to "fix" yourself — and start understanding yourself.

Let's explore how to build this habit of compassionate awareness through practical tools, real-world methods, and reflections that help you connect science with intuition.

Glucose Tracking: Your Metabolic Compass

Glucose monitoring is one of the most powerful ways to understand how your body processes food, stress, and sleep.

You can use a **Continuous Glucose Monitor (CGM)** or a **finger-prick glucometer** to track your blood sugar levels before and after meals, workouts, and rest.

But here's the mindset shift: you're not looking for "good" or "bad" numbers — you're looking for *patterns*.

Every woman's glucose response is unique. A banana may spike one person's blood sugar but barely affect another's. The magic is in observing and adjusting. Over time, your data will teach you how to:

- Time meals around your energy rhythms

- Pair foods to blunt glucose spikes

- Identify which carbs or meals lead to energy crashes

- Recognize how stress, sleep, and movement affect your readings

The goal is not to chase perfection but to build awareness. When you see the connection between what you eat and how you feel — your relationship with food transforms.

How to Track Glucose Effectively

1. Start with Baseline Measurements

Each morning, take a fasting glucose reading — ideally within 15–20 minutes of waking. This gives you a baseline of your metabolic state before food or movement.

2. Pre- and Post-Meal Checks

Take a reading right before eating, then again 60–90 minutes after. You'll see how your body processes that specific meal.

- A gentle rise followed by a steady return to baseline is ideal.

- A sharp spike followed by a crash may indicate poor food pairing or timing.

3. Use Your Journal to Connect the Dots

Write down what you ate, when you ate, and how you felt two hours later. Did you feel focused or fatigued? Calm or anxious? Data becomes meaningful only when connected to experience.

4. Walk It Off

A 10–15 minute walk after meals can significantly lower glucose spikes — not because it burns calories, but because it helps muscles soak up circulating glucose. Think of walking as part of digestion.

5. Weekly Reflection

At the end of each week, note which meals supported your energy best. Which caused swings? This is how you build your personalized "glucose blueprint."

Recommended Tracking Tools

The goal is to make data simple, visible, and meaningful. Below are some of the most user-friendly, science-backed tools to support your Reinvented journey.

1. Withings Body+ or Body Scan Scale

What It Measures:

- Weight, body fat %, muscle mass, visceral fat, and bone density

- Syncs automatically with your phone via the Health Mate app

Why It Matters:

Body composition tells the real story. You may weigh the same, but if your muscle mass rises and your fat mass drops — you're transforming. Withings provides an easy, visual way to track those changes weekly without fixating on the scale.

How to Use It:

- Weigh yourself once a day (to look for weekly trends), same time, same conditions (ideally morning, fasted).

- Track the trend, not the number.

- Look for gradual improvements — consistency beats rapid

change every time.

2. WHOOP Band

What It Measures:

- Recovery, strain, heart rate variability (HRV), and sleep quality

- Tracks how your body responds to workouts, stress, and rest

Why It Matters:

The WHOOP helps you see how well you're balancing effort and recovery. It shows when your body is ready to push harder — and when you need to rest.

How to Use It:

- Review your Recovery Score each morning. A green day? Go lift. A red day? Focus on stretching or a walk.

- Track how caffeine, late meals, or alcohol affect your sleep.

- Use sleep data to fine-tune your bedtime and nightly routine.

3. Continuous Glucose Monitors (CGMs)

Examples: Levels, Nutrisense, Freestyle Libre
What It Measures: Real-time glucose fluctuations throughout the day.

Why It Matters:

Unlike a single reading, CGMs show patterns. You'll see how specific meals, snacks, workouts, and even emotions impact your glucose curve.

How to Use It:

- Wear the sensor for 14 days at a time.

- Log your meals and activities in the app.

- Identify your "trigger foods" (those that cause high spikes or crashes).

- Pair high-carb foods with protein or fat next time — then watch your data respond.

4. RENPHO Tape Measure

What It Measures: Waist, hips, arms, and thighs — digitally synced to your phone.

Why It Matters:

Waist-to-hip ratio is one of the strongest indicators of metabolic health. As you stabilize glucose and build muscle, your waistline often shrinks before the scale moves.

How to Use It:

- Measure every 2 weeks.

- Record your results in your Reinvented Journal.

- Celebrate subtle progress — inches lost often mean inflammation reduced.

The Mindset of Measurement

Tracking is not about being perfect — it's about being present.

Every number you record, every note you make, is an act of awareness. When you track with compassion, you begin to replace judgment with curiosity. You stop asking, "What's wrong with me?" and start asking, "What is my body trying to tell me?"

Data should not drain your joy; it should deepen your understanding.

Some days your glucose will spike. Some weeks your weight won't move. Those are not setbacks — they're signals. They're part of your personal blueprint being revealed.

Weekly Reflection: Turning Data Into Insight

At the end of each week, take a few minutes to review your notes. Ask yourself:

1. Energy Patterns: When did I feel my best? When did I feel low?

2. Meal Awareness: Which foods kept me full and steady? Which caused dips or crashes?

3. Movement Wins: How did exercise affect my sleep, mood, or cravings?

4. Stress Check: Did I notice any link between stress and glucose spikes?

5. Recovery Reality: How many nights this week did I truly rest?

The answers aren't judgments — they're insights. You're not tracking to punish yourself. You're tracking to support yourself.

Bringing It All Together

Here's the bigger picture:

- **Glucose tracking** shows how your metabolism responds in real time.

- **Body composition** shows how your habits shape your physique.

- **Recovery tracking** ensures your body can adapt and thrive.

- **Mindful journaling** integrates emotion, energy, and experience into the data.

When you use all four together, you no longer guess your way to results. You build them — with clarity, with grace, and with science on your side.

Reflection Prompt: The Science of Self-Compassion

Before you move forward, pause and ask yourself:

- What data points tend to trigger frustration for me — and why?

- How can I view them as neutral feedback instead of personal failure?

- What's one way I can make tracking feel nurturing instead of stressful?

- How will I celebrate consistency instead of perfection this week?

Because this journey isn't about perfection — it's about precision.

Not discipline — but devotion.
Not control — but connection.

Closing Note

The *Reinvented* approach to tracking is about grace in motion. It's not about chasing numbers or hacking biology — it's about honoring the elegant design of your body.

When you understand how your glucose, hormones, sleep, and movement interact, you stop fighting yourself. You begin to lead yourself.

Science gives you the framework. Awareness gives you the freedom.

Together, they give you the power to live Reinvented.

Chapter 12:
Resources: Putting Science And Self Care Into Action

The Science Behind Reinvented

A Woman's Health Blueprint, Grounded in Research and Redefined for Real Life

Every recommendation in **Reinvented** is built on decades of clinical research — but more importantly, it's built around you.

For too long, weight loss has been treated as a numbers game. But the science now confirms what most women already feel intuitively: **health is about composition, not just scale weight.** How much of your body is strong, metabolically active muscle versus stored fat determines your energy, balance, and vitality — not the number flashing on the scale.

The science of *Reinvented* shifts the focus from *restriction* to *restoration* — helping you rebuild your strength, metabolism, and confidence at every stage of womanhood.

1. Why the Scale Isn't the Whole Story

Most traditional weight-loss plans cause your body to lose both fat and lean muscle — and that matters.

Studies show that **20–40% of the weight lost** in conventional dieting comes from lean tissue like muscle, not fat. That loss weakens metabolism, drains energy, and accelerates aging.

Even worse, repeated cycles of dieting and regaining can lead to a condition called **sarcopenic obesity** — when muscle mass decreases while fat increases, leaving the body weaker and metabolically sluggish.

> **What this means for you:**
> The goal isn't just to lose weight. It's to protect your muscle — your body's built-in fat-burning engine.

2. A New Definition of "Healthy Weight"

Clinicians now recommend measuring progress by body composition rather than pounds alone. Waist circumference, muscle quality, and blood sugar stability matter far more than BMI.

Research shows that even a **5–15% reduction in body weight** can improve blood sugar, cholesterol, and blood pressure — especially when that weight comes primarily from fat loss, not muscle loss.

> **In other words:** small, consistent improvements change your entire metabolic future.

3. Protein: Your Body's Best Investment

Among all macronutrients, **protein takes center stage** in body recomposition.

Clinical studies show that consuming **1.2–1.6 grams per kilogram** of body weight — or roughly **0.55–0.73 grams per pound** — each day helps preserve lean muscle, support hormone balance, and stabilize glucose during weight loss.

Protein isn't just for athletes — it's for every woman who wants to stay strong, clear-headed, and hormonally balanced.

> **Real takeaway:** eat enough high-quality protein (fish, eggs, lean meats, or plant-based blends) to keep your body in "rebuild" mode, not "breakdown" mode.

4. Carbs, Glucose, and Hormonal Balance

Here's where the science gets exciting: your blood sugar rhythm affects everything — your energy, mood, cravings, and hormones.

Studies show that women who stabilize glucose (by pairing carbs with protein and fiber, and walking after meals) experience less fatigue, better focus, and fewer hormonal swings.

> **Simple fix:** manage glucose, and your metabolism naturally resets itself.
> No deprivation, no extremes — just timing, balance, and awareness.

5. Exercise: The Sculptor of Strength

Research is clear: **resistance training changes everything.** When you combine resistance with aerobic exercise, your body learns to lose fat while keeping muscle.

Clinical data on women show:

- Lower-body strength can improve by 7% per week with consistent resistance training.

- Upper-body strength follows closely behind at around 5%.

- Combining strength and cardio doubles results in fat loss and muscle tone.

Even walking for 10–15 minutes after meals helps regulate glucose and enhance fat metabolism.

> **Movement tip:** you don't need hours in the gym — just consistent effort, and a mix of strength + steady movement.

6. Modern Medicine Meets Metabolic Science

For some women, **GLP-1 receptor agonists** (like semaglutide or tirzepatide) can enhance results when combined with lifestyle change.
These medications mimic natural hormones that improve glucose control, slow digestion, and increase fullness — leading to weight loss without muscle sacrifice.

However, research makes one thing clear: **these tools work best when paired with protein-rich meals, resistance training, and healthy sleep.**

> **Bottom line:** modern medicine can support your body's design — but it can't replace it.

7. The Power of Whole-Person Care

Long-term health isn't achieved in isolation.
The most successful programs combine nutrition, movement, medical insight, and emotional support. Teams of physicians, dietitians, and fitness professionals now collaborate to personalize plans for women's unique metabolic needs.

Ongoing monitoring of glucose, muscle mass, and energy levels helps sustain progress.

> **Because health isn't a destination — it's a rhythm your body learns to trust.**

Let's Break It Down

Here's the simple truth behind all of it:

When you **feed your body the right fuel, move with purpose, and stabilize your glucose**, you naturally shift toward a healthier, more balanced version of yourself.

Your body learns to:

- Preserve muscle instead of burning it

- Use fat for fuel

- Maintain steady energy

- Balance hormones naturally

It's not about dieting harder.
It's about working *smarter* — with your biology, not against it.

So take a breath. Pour a glass of water (or your favorite matcha). And let's put all this research into real, everyday action — designed for your body, your lifestyle, and your next chapter.

Summary of Key Studies on Women, Glucose, and Body Transformation

Here's what the science says — made simple and practical.

1 Weight Loss + Exercise Preserves Muscle
Women ages 45–65 who added exercise (especially strength training) to calorie restriction kept their muscle while losing fat.
☞ *Takeaway: Always include resistance training — diet alone costs muscle.*

2 Resistance + Cardio = Best Results
Postmenopausal women saw the best body composition changes when combining both aerobic and strength workouts.
☞ *Walk or cycle for fat loss, lift for tone and strength.*

3 Women Build Strength Quickly
Studies show lower-body strength can increase by 7% per week with consistent effort.
☞ *Visible results start in weeks, not years.*

4 Higher Volume Helps Post-Menopause
More sets and reps led to stronger, more muscular bodies in postmenopausal women.
☞ *Don't scale back — increase volume mindfully.*

5 Smart Weight Loss Protects Muscle
Combining resistance + cardio while eating enough protein prevents lean mass loss.

☞ *Nutrition + training = muscle protection.*

6 Small Weight Loss = Big Glucose Gains
Even 5–10% body weight loss improved insulin sensitivity and stabilized glucose.

☞ *Progress over perfection — small wins matter.*

7 GLP-1 Hormones Support Appetite Control
These hormones (naturally or via medication) improve satiety and stabilize glucose.

☞ *Protein and fiber meals mimic this naturally.*

8 Sleep & Stress Are Glucose Regulators
One poor night of sleep can spike glucose the next day.

☞ *Recovery and rest are as essential as reps.*

Modern wellness isn't about chasing numbers — it's about understanding what your body truly needs to thrive. *Reinvented* translates decades of research into a blueprint that honors the unique physiology of women across every stage of life.

The New Science of Strength

Traditional weight loss often causes women to lose as much muscle as fat. Studies show that up to 40% of total weight lost in standard diets can come from metabolically active muscle — the very tissue that keeps our energy high and metabolism strong.

> "Weight loss should never come at
> the expense of strength."
> — *Reinvented Research Summary, 2024*

Instead, Reinvented redefines the goal:
Reduce fat mass, protect muscle, and rebuild metabolic vitality.

Fuel That Works With You, Not Against You

Protein is more than a macronutrient — it's the foundation of renewal. Research suggests women benefit most from 1.2–1.6g of protein per kilogram of body weight daily to maintain muscle during transformation.

Quality matters as much as quantity. Lean fish, eggs, chicken, and whey isolate provide essential amino acids like leucine — the "spark plug" of muscle protein synthesis.

> "Nourish to flourish — your body is not
> meant to be starved, but supported."

Move With Intention

Science confirms that the type of exercise matters as much as consistency.
A blend of resistance and aerobic training is the most powerful formula for fat loss, hormone balance, and longevity.

Resistance training preserves muscle and builds bone density — crucial for women entering perimenopause and beyond. Aerobic movement, from brisk walks to cycling, enhances fat metabolism and cardiovascular health.

> "Movement is medicine — and resistance is its prescription."

Even 10 minutes of walking after meals can help regulate blood glucose, improve energy, and support a calmer nervous system.

Metabolic Support Meets Modern Science

For some women, medical therapies such as GLP-1 receptor agonists can complement lifestyle changes. These tools, when prescribed responsibly, help regulate appetite, balance insulin response, and sustain long-term progress — always as part of a holistic plan that centers lifestyle first.

> "Modern medicine can support nature's design — not replace it."

Whole-Woman Wellness

The research behind *Reinvented* emphasizes one clear truth: Women's health cannot be reduced to a number on a scale.

By protecting lean muscle, balancing hormones, and supporting a flexible metabolism, women can create health that is *visible, vibrant, and sustainable.*

> "The goal isn't smaller. The goal is stronger."

The Reinvented Equation

Nutrition + Movement + Mindful Science = Sustainable Energy & Lifelong Strength

This integrated approach honors your body as a living system — one that deserves nourishment, balance, and respect at every age.

Through evidence, intention, and daily practice, *Reinvented* transforms data into daily ritual — helping women not just understand the science, but *live* it.

Chapter 13:
Meal Timing Framework:
Fat Loss → Maintenance

This isn't about restriction—it's about *reinvention*.

By aligning when you eat with how your hormones work, you lower cortisol, stabilize glucose, and unlock fat burning while protecting muscle.

Phase 1: Fat Loss Reset

Two Meals Per Day + Optional "Workout-Snacks" (A workout-snack is NOT food, it's 10 minutes of exercise - like walking, squats, lunges, pushups, etc. Work-out snacks throughout the day means you're moving more.)

- **Meal 1 (Breakfast): Eat within 15–20 minutes of waking up.**

    ○ Why: Skipping breakfast in midlife often backfires. Without fuel, cortisol rises, glucose spikes, and cravings hit later. A protein-rich breakfast sets the stage for stable energy and fat loss.

    ○ Example: Protein smoothie with chia + berries OR tofu scramble with spinach + avocado.

- **Pre/Post-"Workout Snack" (Optional):**

  - Small, protein-based snack if you train in the morning (e.g., hard-boiled egg, handful of edamame, or half a protein shake).

  - Post-workout: Walk 10–15 minutes after to blunt glucose spikes.

- **Meal 2 ("Linner"): 5–6 hours later.**

  - Why: Extending the window between meals reduces glucose excursions, improves insulin sensitivity, and gives your body time to fully digest before sleep.

  - Example: Lentil + chickpea bowl with veggies and tahini, or salmon + roasted vegetables with quinoa.

- **Evening: No dinner during the fat-loss phase. Hydrate, sip herbal tea, and prepare for consistent sleep.**

  - Why: Going to bed with stable glucose allows fat burning to dominate overnight.

Phase 2: Maintenance Lifestyle

Three Meals Per Day

Once you've reached your goal weight or body fat percentage, you can reintroduce dinner—with strategy:

- Keep dinner earlier (at least 3–4 hours before bedtime).

- Stick to glucose-friendly pairings (protein + veggies first, carbs last).

- Use glucose rhythm rituals when enjoying splurges (exercise after eating, cinnamon, vinegar, protein-first sequencing).

Why It Works

- **Cortisol Control:** Morning fuel prevents stress-driven glucose spikes.

- **Glucose Stability:** Two balanced meals = fewer daily spikes, more fat burning.

- **Fat Burning at Night:** Going to bed with low glucose encourages fat as a fuel source while you sleep.

- **Flexibility:** Adding dinner back during maintenance makes this a lifestyle, not a diet.

Mindset Shift: Restriction → Reinvention

This approach isn't about deprivation. You can enjoy splurges when you want, but you'll know how to blunt their effects and keep your body composition steady. By learning how to control glucose, you're free from yo-yo dieting and calorie obsession.

> **You're not just eating less. You're eating *smarter*, aligned with your hormones and metabolism.**

Meal Templates + Glucose-Friendly Recipes

Guiding Principles for Glucose-Friendly Meals

- **Protein First:** Aim for 25–30g protein per meal (goal: ~1g per pound of body weight daily).

- **Veggies for Volume:** Fill half your plate with non-starchy vegetables.

- **Carbs Strategically:** Choose whole-food carbs (beans, lentils, quinoa, oats, fruit) and pair with protein/fiber.

- **Healthy Fats as Stabilizers:** Avocado, nuts, seeds, olive oil, tahini = glucose brakes.

- **Meal Sequencing:** Eat protein-first, carbs last for lower glucose readings.

Meal Template 1: Breakfast (Protein + Fiber + Healthy Fat)

- **Plant-Based Option:**

    - Overnight oats with chia seeds, hemp seeds, almond butter, and unsweetened soy milk

    - Topped with berries (fiber + antioxidants)

- **Animal Protein Add-On:**

    - Greek yogurt or whey protein mixed in for extra protein boost

- Why it works: Oats + chia provide slow-release carbs, while seeds and nut butter lower the effects of glucose.

Meal Template 2: Lunch (Protein + Colorful Veg + Whole Carb)

- **Plant-Based Option:**

    - Lentil + chickpea salad with spinach, cucumbers, bell peppers, olive oil, and lemon dressing

    - Side of quinoa or roasted sweet potato

- **Animal Protein Add-On:**

    - Grilled salmon, chicken breast, or boiled eggs on top

- Why it works: Lentils and chickpeas give fiber + plant protein, with healthy fats from olive oil slowing glucose rise.

Meal Template 3: Dinner (Protein + Roasted Veg + Optional Grain)

- **Plant-Based Option:**

    - Tofu or tempeh stir-fry with broccoli, bok choy, mushrooms, garlic, and tamari sauce

    - Serve over cauliflower rice or quinoa

- **Animal Protein Add-On:**

    - Shrimp, lean beef, or roasted turkey breast

- Why it works: High protein, fiber-rich veggies, and moderate carbs for balanced glucose response.

Meal Template 4: Snacks (Protein + Fiber)

- **Plant-Based Option:**

  - Apple slices with almond butter

  - Roasted edamame or chickpeas

  - Veggies + hummus

- **Animal Protein Add-On:**

  - Hard-boiled egg or turkey roll-ups

- Why it works: Protein + fiber keeps you fuller, reduces cravings, and prevents spikes from snacking on high-carb foods alone.

Glucose-Friendly Recipes

Protein-Packed Lentil Bowl

Ingredients:

- 1 cup cooked green lentils

- 1 cup roasted vegetables (zucchini, peppers, carrots)

- 2 tbsp tahini

- 1 tbsp olive oil

- Handful of arugula or spinach

- Squeeze of lemon

Animal Protein Option: Top with grilled chicken or salmon.

Why It Works: Lentils are high in fiber + protein, veggies add volume, and tahini + olive oil provide healthy fats to blunt glucose rise.

Tofu + Veggie Stir-Fry with Cauliflower Rice

Ingredients:

- 1 block firm tofu, cubed

- 2 cups broccoli, snap peas, and mushrooms

- 2 cloves garlic, minced

- 1 tbsp sesame oil

- 2 tbsp low-sodium tamari

- Serve over cauliflower rice

Animal Protein Option: Replace tofu with shrimp or chicken breast.

Why It Works: High protein + fiber + low glycemic carb base keeps glucose steady.

Chia Protein Pudding

Ingredients:

- 3 tbsp chia seeds

- 1 cup unsweetened almond or soy milk

- 1 scoop plant-based protein powder (pea or hemp)

- 1 tsp cinnamon (helps lower glucose response)

- Top with blueberries + walnuts

Animal Protein Option: Swap plant protein for whey or collagen powder.

Why It Works: High protein, high fiber, healthy fat = steady energy and no crash.

Chapter 14: Sample Resistance + HIIT Training Programs by Age & Level

Women in Their 40s: Building & Preserving Muscle

Focus: Strength + Glucose Sensitivity + Bone Density

Beginner (2 strength + 2 HIIT/week)

- Strength: 2 days (e.g., Mon/Thu) HIIT: 2 sessions (10–15 min, Tue/Fri)
    - 20-sec fast walk / 100-sec easy walk × 5 rounds
- Example Strength Day:
    - Squats (bodyweight → goblet) — 3x12
    - Push-ups (incline → floor) — 3x8–10
    - Rows (bands or dumbbells) — 3x12
    - Glute bridges — 3x12

Intermediate (3 strength + 2 HIIT/week)

- Strength: Mon/Wed/Fri
- HIIT: Tue/Sat (10–12 min)
    - 30-sec sprint / 90-sec recovery × 5
- Example: Deadlifts, push-ups, split squats, overhead press.

Advanced (3–4 strength + 2 HIIT/week)

- Strength: Mon/Tue/Thu/Sat
- HIIT: Wed/Sun (10–15 min)
    - Bike sprints: 20-sec all-out / 2-min recovery × 5
- Example: Barbell squats, pull-ups, deadlifts, bench press.

Women in Their 50s: Strength for Hormone Harmony

Focus: Preserve Lean Mass + Bone Strength + Glucose Stability

Beginner (2 strength + 2 HIIT/week)

- Strength: 2 days (Mon/Thu)
- HIIT: 2 days (Tue/Fri)
    - Hill walking or bike: 30-sec push / 2-min recovery × 4–5

Intermediate (3 strength + 2 HIIT/week)

- Strength: Mon/Wed/Fri
- HIIT: Tue/Sat (12 min)
    - Rowing machine or elliptical: 40-sec hard / 80-sec recovery × 6

Advanced (3 strength + 2 HIIT/week)

- Strength: Mon/Wed/Fri
- HIIT: Thu/Sun (15 min)
    - Sprint/walk intervals: 30-sec sprint / 90-sec walk × 6–7
- Strength Example: Hip thrusts, squats, pull-ups, bench press.

Women 60+: Staying Strong, Mobile, & Independent

Focus: Functional Strength + Balance + Longevity

Beginner (2 strength + 2 HIIT/week)

- Strength: 2 days (Tue/Fri)
- HIIT: 2 days (Mon/Thu, 8–10 min)
    - Gentle intervals: 20-sec brisk walk / 90-sec slow walk × 4–5

Intermediate (2–3 strength + 2 HIIT/week)

- Strength: Mon/Wed/Fri
- HIIT: Tue/Sat (10–12 min)
    - Stationary bike: 20-sec push / 100-sec recovery × 5

Advanced (3 strength + 2 HIIT/week)

- Strength: Mon/Wed/Fri
- HIIT: Thu/Sun (12–15 min)
    - Power walk with incline or rowing machine: 30-sec strong / 90-sec recovery × 6

Programming Notes

- **HIIT = Short & Sweet:** 10–15 minutes max, 2x/week only.

- **Pairing Strategy:** Never do HIIT + heavy strength on the same day unless short on time (if combined, keep HIIT after strength).

- **Balance Hormones:** Too much HIIT raises cortisol—2x/week is the sweet spot for fat loss, insulin sensitivity, and heart health.

- **Recovery Matters:** Alternate HIIT + strength days when possible; rest or mobility work on Sundays if energy feels low.

Quick-Start 1-Day Meal + Workout Schedule

Phase: Fat Loss Reset (2 meals/day + optional workout snack)
Goal: Stabilize glucose, build/maintain muscle, and optimize fat burning overnight.

Morning (Within 15–20 Minutes of Waking)

- **Meal 1: Protein-Heavy Breakfast**

    - **Plant-Based:** Chia protein pudding with soy milk, blueberries, hemp seeds

    - **Animal Add-On:** 2 boiled eggs or scoop of whey protein

- **Why:** Blunts morning cortisol, stabilizes glucose, sets the tone for fat burning.

If Training in the Morning:

- Have a **small protein snack** (half shake, handful of edamame, or 1 boiled egg) before.

- Do **strength training or HIIT** (20–40 min).

- **Walk 10–15 minutes afterward** to blunt glucose spike.

Midday–Afternoon (5–6 Hours Later)

- **Meal 2: "Linner" (Lunch + Dinner Combo)**

    - ○ **Plant-Based:** Lentil & chickpea salad with spinach, cucumbers, tahini, olive oil

    - ○ **Animal Add-On:** Grilled salmon or chicken breast

    - ○ **Side:** Quinoa or roasted sweet potato

- **Why:** Long gap between meals improves insulin sensitivity and allows full digestion before bed.

- **If Training in the Afternoon:**

- Do strength training session 1–2 hours before Linner.

- Follow with post-meal walk (10–15 min).

Evening

- No heavy dinner during fat loss phase.

- Hydrate with water or herbal tea.

- Light mobility work, stretching, or a calming walk.

Bedtime Routine

- Aim for **7–9 hours of sleep.**

- Keep last meal at least 3–4 hours before bed.

- Create a "wind-down" ritual (no screens, dim lights, read or journal).

Why: Stable glucose overnight = fat burning + hormone reset while you sleep.

Daily Quick-Start Recap

- Eat protein within 20 min of waking

- Strength or HIIT + post-workout walk

- One large balanced "Linner" 5–6 hrs later

- Evening fasting window until next morning

- Sleep early = fat burn + recovery

3-Day Fat Loss Phase Sample Plan

Framework:

- **Meal 1:** Within 15–20 minutes of waking (protein-rich).

- **Meal 2 ("Linner"):** 5–6 hours later (large, balanced).

- **No Dinner:** Herbal tea, hydration, light mobility in evening.

- **Movement:** Strength training 2–3x/week, HIIT 2x/week, walks after meals.

Day 1: Strength + Steady Energy

Breakfast (7:00 AM)

- Chia protein pudding with soy milk, hemp seeds, blueberries

- **Add-on:** 2 boiled eggs or scoop whey protein
  Fuels muscles + blunts cortisol spike

Workout (8:00 AM)

- Strength Training (Lower Body Focus)

    o Squats — 3x10

    o Glute bridges — 3x12

    o Step-ups — 3x10 per leg

    o Band rows — 3x12

- Post-workout: 10-min walk

Linner (1:00 PM)

- Lentil + chickpea salad with cucumbers, spinach, tahini

- **Add-on:** Grilled salmon or chicken breast
  Large, balanced meal with protein + fiber + healthy fat

Evening

- Herbal tea, stretching, foam rolling

- Bed by 10:00 PM

Day 2: HIIT + Hormone Reset

Breakfast (6:45 AM)

- Protein smoothie: unsweetened soy milk, pea protein, spinach, chia, ½ banana

- **Add-on:** Scoop collagen or whey for extra protein

Workout (7:30 AM)

- HIIT (Bike or Brisk Walk Intervals)

    o 30 sec sprint / 90 sec recovery × 5

- Post-HIIT: 10-min easy walk to lower glucose

Linner (12:30 PM)

- Tofu stir-fry with broccoli, mushrooms, bok choy, sesame oil

- **Add-on:** Shrimp or lean beef strips

- **Side:** Cauliflower rice or quinoa

Evening

- Light walk after dinner time (even though no meal)

- Guided meditation for stress reset

- Sleep 7–9 hours

Day 3: Full Body Strength + Long Fasting Window

Breakfast (7:30 AM)

- Oatmeal with chia, flax, almond butter, cinnamon

- **Add-on:** Greek yogurt or protein powder stirred in
  High-fiber + high-protein start = lower glucose readings

Workout (9:00 AM)

- Strength Training (Full Body)

  - Deadlifts — 3x8

  - Push-ups — 3x8–10

  - Bulgarian split squats — 3x8 per leg

  - Overhead press — 3x10

- Post-workout: 10–15 min walk

Linner (2:00 PM)

- Quinoa bowl with black beans, roasted zucchini, bell peppers, olive oil

- **Add-on:** Grilled chicken or turkey slices
  Protein + Whole Food base, long satiety, stable glucose

Evening

- Herbal tea, journaling or reading

- In bed by 9:30–10:00 PM

Fat Loss Phase Keys

- **2 Meals/Day:** Protein-heavy breakfast + large linner 5–6 hrs later.

- **Workouts:** Alternate strength and HIIT, with walks post-meals.

- **Evening Fast:** No dinner during fat-loss phase → stable overnight glucose + fat burning.

- **Consistency > Perfection:** Adjust timing to your lifestyle, but keep the principles: protein, glucose-friendly pairings, movement.

Resources: From Knowledge to Action

You've reached the end of the resources section, and now you have everything you need to turn science into practice. The studies have shown us the truth: women in midlife can *gain muscle, burn fat, and transform their bodies* at any age when the right strategies are in place.

You've seen the tools:

- **Meal Templates + Recipes** — practical ways to keep glucose steady while enjoying satisfying food.

- **Meal Timing Framework** — two meals a day during fat loss to lower glucose and unlock overnight fat burning, with flexibility for maintenance.

- **Sample Training Programs** — resistance workouts + HIIT tailored by age and level, proving strength is possible (and essential) at every stage.

- **Tools and Tracking Worksheets** — simple tools to help you connect the dots between food, glucose, hormones, stress, and results.

- **3-Day Sample Plan** — a plug-and-play roadmap showing exactly how to pair meals and workouts for fat loss.

Your Transformation, Your Blueprint

What makes this different from every diet and program out there? It's **yours**. This isn't about following rigid rules, endless cardio, or starving yourself. It's about building a lifestyle where:

- Glucose is steady.

- Muscle is strong.

- Sleep is restorative.

- Stress is managed.

- Food is nourishing, not restrictive.

This isn't about shrinking yourself—it's about **rebuilding yourself**.

Your Call to Action

Now it's your turn. Take the first step:

- Print the worksheets.

- Choose a meal template for tomorrow's breakfast.

- Block out two days for strength training this week.

- Commit to one glucose-friendly habit (protein first, exercise after eating, or earlier bedtime).

Small actions, repeated consistently, will transform your body and your life.

Your Call to Action

Now it's your turn. Take the first step:

- Print the worksheets.

- Choose a meal template for tomorrow's breakfast.

- Block out two days for strength training this week.

- Commit to one glucose-friendly habit (protein first, exercise after eating, or earlier bedtime).

Small actions, repeated consistently, will transform your body and your life.

Looking Ahead

This book was the framework. These resources are the tools. The next step is you living it—choosing, experimenting, tracking, adjusting, and celebrating your progress.

You don't need perfection. You need **progress**.
You don't need restriction. You need **reinvention**.

This is your blueprint. This is your body. This is your next chapter.

"Transformation doesn't begin with a diet or a deadline — it begins the moment you decide to know yourself better."

— Unknown

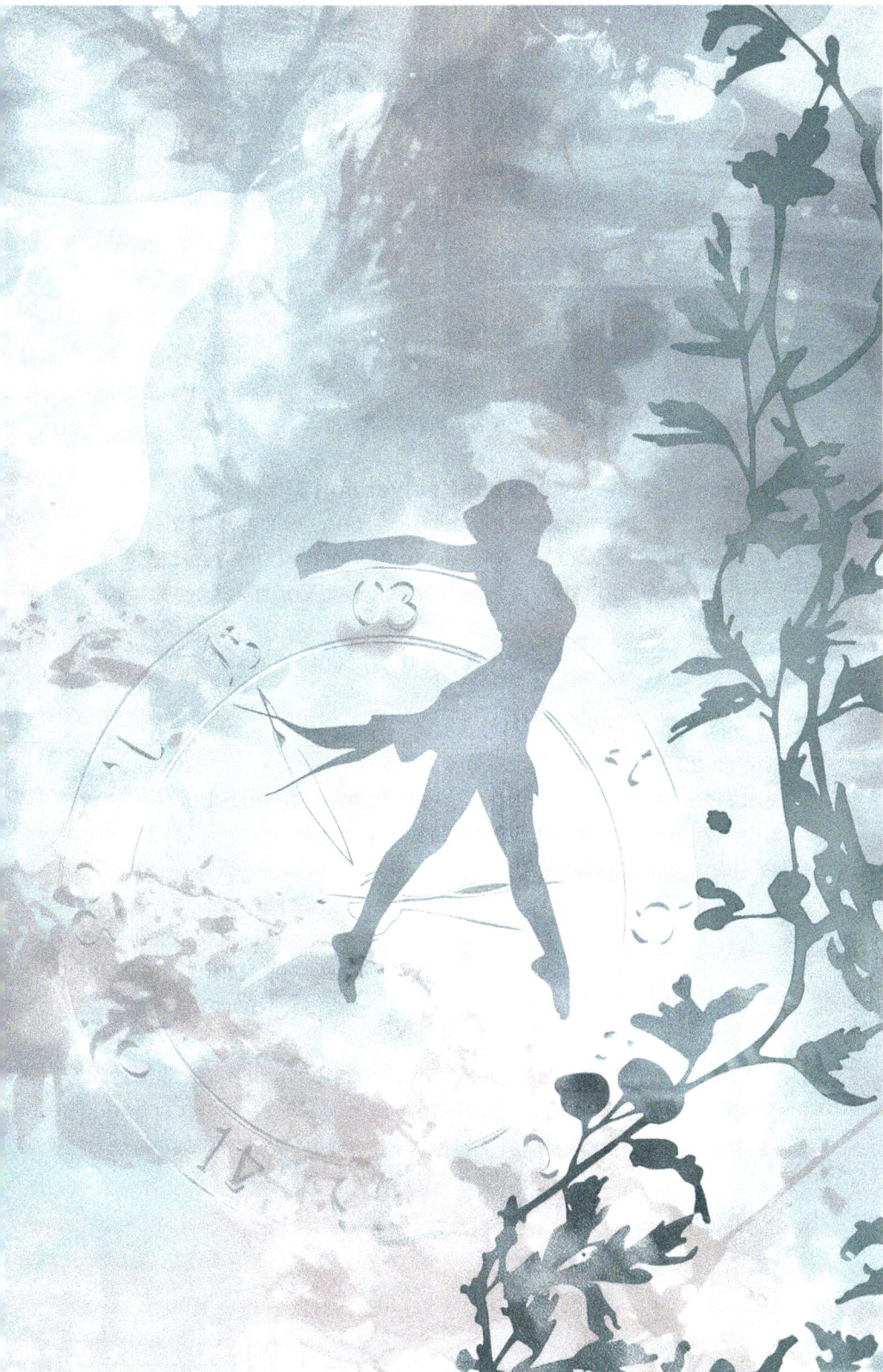

Chapter 15:
The Reinvention Mindset

The R.E.S.E.T. Method

A daily framework for real, lasting change.

Once you understand the **Reinvention Mindset**, it's time to bring it to life through daily action — one choice, one meal, one movement at a time. Transformation isn't built overnight; it's created through rhythm, awareness, and consistency.

That's where the **R.E.S.E.T. Method** comes in.

This framework was designed to make the science of glucose balance and hormone harmony simple, tangible, and repeatable. It's not about perfection or restriction — it's about giving your body the environment it needs to thrive.

Each letter in **R.E.S.E.T.** represents a small, science-backed habit that stabilizes your glucose, lowers cortisol, and supports fat loss while preserving muscle. These are the daily rituals that bring balance back to your metabolism and energy back to your life.

You won't need to memorize complex meal plans or follow rigid schedules. Instead, you'll learn to listen, adjust, and respond to your body — using tools that teach you what works best for you.

Over time, this becomes second nature — a graceful rhythm of nourishment, movement, and self-awareness that anchors your day and reshapes your health from the inside out.

Because reinvention isn't just about big moments of change.

It's about the quiet discipline of small steps done with purpose — the kind that lead to balance, confidence, and strength that lasts.

The R.E.S.E.T. Method

A simple system for stabilizing glucose, balancing hormones, and restoring energy.

R — Record Your Numbers
Start by knowing your body.
Track your glucose throughout the day — before and after meals, and at bedtime. Notice how your food, stress, and movement affect your levels. Awareness creates clarity, and clarity creates change.

E — Eat Early
Your body runs on rhythm.
Eating within 15–30 minutes of waking helps regulate cortisol and prevents an early glucose spike. This sets the tone for steadier energy, better focus, and smoother digestion all day long. Also, finish your last meal earlier in the evening to allow your body time to process glucose and gently return to fat-burning mode before sleep — supporting deeper rest, balanced hormones, and overnight recovery.

S — Sequence Food Order

How you eat matters as much as what you eat.

Start meals with protein and fiber, add healthy fats next, and finish with carbohydrates. This order slows glucose absorption and supports sustained energy. A small "pre-meal ritual" — like apple cider vinegar or a few squats — can further blunt spikes.

E — Exercise After Eating

Movement is medicine.

A simple 10–15 minute walk or light resistance workout after meals helps your muscles absorb glucose for energy instead of storing it as fat. Think of it as closing the loop between nourishment and motion.

T — Target Under 100 by Bedtime

Your evening number sets the stage for recovery.

When glucose is below 100 before bed, your body shifts into fat-burning and repair mode while you sleep. It's your nightly reset — the quiet magic of metabolic balance.

Every day you R.E.S.E.T., you realign with your body's natural intelligence.

You build balance, one choice at a time — and that's where reinvention truly begins.

Reflect + Reinvent: Your Daily RESET Practice

Turn awareness into action, and action into balance.

Now that you understand the **R.E.S.E.T. Method**, it's time to make it your own.

The power of this framework doesn't come from perfection — it comes from presence.
These prompts are here to help you observe your body, your energy, and your progress with compassion, not criticism.

Each day is an opportunity to listen more deeply and respond more wisely — to reconnect with the intelligence your body already has.

Take a few quiet minutes to reflect, either in the morning as you set your intention or at night as you review your day.

A Letter to the Woman You're Becoming

There's a quiet moment — sometime after the last diet, the last scale check, the last "I'll start again Monday" — when you finally exhale and realize you don't need to fight your body anymore. You just need to understand it.

That's where reinvention begins.

It's not a dramatic overnight transformation or a race toward perfection. It's a gradual unfolding — a returning — to the body that's been with you through every version of your life.
The one that carried your laughter, your heartbreak, your resilience, your wins, and your lessons.
The one that never gave up on you.

Redefining Strength

You've learned that strength isn't found in restriction, but in rhythm.
It's in the decision to nourish instead of punish.
To train because you can, not because you should.
To rest not out of guilt, but out of wisdom.

Strong isn't a look — it's a feeling.
It's walking into your day steady and self-assured.
It's choosing foods that love you back.
It's trusting your body again.

When you treat strength as sacred, your body responds with grace.

Redefining Balance

Balance is no longer something you chase — it's something you cultivate.
It's in the morning walk that resets your glucose.
The quiet moment of breath before a meal.
The eight hours of sleep that become non-negotiable because your energy is worth protecting.

Balance doesn't mean doing it all — it means doing what matters most.
And sometimes, that means saying no to chaos and yes to calm.

Redefining Beauty

There's a special kind of beauty that arrives when you stop trying to be younger — and start trying to be well.
When you stop shrinking yourself — in body, in voice, in ambition — and start expanding into your full, radiant power.
That's the beauty of reinvention.

It's confidence rooted in chemistry.
It's elegance powered by energy.
It's the knowing that health and happiness are not separate goals — they are the same destination.

Redefining Success

Success isn't measured in pounds or perfection.
It's in waking up with energy that lasts.
It's in clarity of mind, peaceful digestion, deep sleep, and genuine joy.
It's in the ability to move through life with more ease, less urgency, and a steady heart.

You've learned to see data not as judgment, but as direction.
To make your tools — glucose monitor, scale, tracker — work for you, not against you.
You've learned that progress is not linear, and that healing never happens in a straight line.

Reinvented — and Still Becoming

Reinvention isn't a finish line.
It's a lifelong conversation between you and your body — one grounded in curiosity, not criticism.
Every walk, every meal, every breath is another chance to listen, adjust, and honor the body that's always been on your side.

You are — and always have been — Reinvented.
Not because you became someone new,
but because you finally remembered who you were all along.

Chapter 16: Journals

This journal is your daily companion—a guide to understanding how your body responds to food, movement, and lifestyle. By tracking your glucose throughout the day, you'll discover your unique baseline and learn how to nourish your body while still enjoying the foods you love (within healthy, mindful boundaries).

Think of this as your starting point for transformation—a tool to help you understand how to lose fat, build or maintain lean muscle, and support your metabolism as you move through your body's natural evolution.

A Note on Commitment

Journaling isn't forever.
We recommend using this tracker for at least **30 days** to observe trends, make adjustments, and identify the ideal blueprint for your body.

Morning Routine

Within **15 minutes of waking**, take your first glucose reading to see where you are starting the day. Then, have breakfast.

Pair **protein and fat with your carbohydrates** to slow glucose absorption and prevent a mid-morning crash. If you plan to work out soon, a light snack—like a few bites of oatmeal with berries and nuts, or yogurt with fruit—is enough to fuel your body and keep cortisol (your stress hormone) from spiking.

After breakfast, take a **10–15 minute walk** to help your body process the meal smoothly.

Midday Check-In

About **three hours later**, take another glucose reading. Has your number returned to <30 from your first reading/baseline? Is it 100 or below? If not, review your breakfast. Try swapping out high-sugar or refined carbs for more **protein, healthy fats, and fiber** next time.

Linner (2–4 PM)

During your fat-burning phase, you'll enjoy two main meals each day: **Breakfast** and **"Linner"** (your late lunch/early dinner).

Before eating, you can check your glucose again to see if your body has returned to fat-burning range. *Linner* should be your **largest meal**—balanced with lean protein, healthy fats, and quality carbohydrates. Eat slowly and stop when you feel **80% full**; this helps train your body to respond naturally to hunger and satisfaction cues.

Glucose-Smart Habits

Before you eat:

- Drink a glass of water with a teaspoon of apple cider vinegar.

- Do a 5–10 minute "exercise snack" (light resistance moves or squats) to activate your muscles—they'll absorb glucose more efficiently at your next meal.

After you eat:

- Take a **10–15 minute walk** to help your glucose levels return to balance.

Evening Wind-Down

After *Linner*, you're done eating until breakfast. Remember: each bite restarts your glucose clock, pulling you out of fat-burning mode.

Check your glucose again **3–4 hours after *Linner*** to see how your body responded to the meal.

Before bed—around **8–10 hours after *Linner***—take a final reading. Ideally, your glucose should be **below 100**, and best in the **80–90 range**, signaling that your body is ready to burn fat overnight.

Then, rest. Sleep is your body's most powerful recovery tool.

Journals

This journal is your daily companion—a guide to understanding how your body responds to food, movement, and lifestyle. By tracking your glucose throughout the day, you'll discover your unique baseline and learn how to nourish your body while still enjoying the foods you love (within healthy, mindful boundaries). Think of this as your starting point for transformation—a tool to help you understand how to lose fat, build or maintain lean muscle, and support your metabolism as you move through your body's natural evolution.

A Note on Commitment

Journaling isn't forever.
We recommend using this tracker for at least 30 days to observe trends, make adjustments, and identify the ideal blueprint for your body.

Morning Routine

Within **15 minutes of waking**, take your first glucose reading to see where you are starting the day. Then, have breakfast.

Pair **protein and fat with your carbohydrates** to slow glucose absorption and prevent a mid-morning crash. If you plan to work out soon, a light snack—like a few bites of oatmeal with berries and nuts, or yogurt with fruit—is enough to fuel your body and keep cortisol (your stress hormone) from spiking.

After breakfast, take a **10–15 minute walk** to help your body process the meal smoothly.

Midday Check-In

About **three hours later**, take another glucose reading. Has your number returned to <30 from your first reading/baseline? Is it 100 or below? If not, review your breakfast. Try swapping out high-sugar or refined carbs for more **protein, healthy fats, and fiber** next time.

Linner (2–4 PM)

During your fat-burning phase, you'll enjoy two main meals each day: **Breakfast** and **"Linner"** (your late lunch/early dinner).

Before eating, you can check your glucose again to see if your body has returned to fat-burning range. Linner should be your **largest meal**—balanced with lean protein, healthy fats, and quality carbohydrates. Eat slowly and stop when you feel **80% full**; this helps train your body to respond naturally to hunger and satisfaction cues.

Glucose-Smart Habits

Before you eat:

- Drink a glass of water with a teaspoon of apple cider vinegar.

- Do a 5–10 minute "exercise snack" (light resistance moves or squats) to activate your muscles—they'll absorb glucose more efficiently at your next meal.

After you eat:

- Take a **10–15 minute walk** to help your glucose levels return to balance.

Evening Wind-Down

After *Linner*, you're done eating until breakfast. Remember: each bite restarts your glucose clock, pulling you out of fat-burning mode.

Check your glucose again **3–4 hours after *Linner*** to see how your body responded to the meal.

Before bed—around **8–10 hours after *Linner***—take a final reading. Ideally, your glucose should be **below 100**, and best in the **80–90 range**, signaling that your body is ready to burn fat overnight.

Then, rest. Sleep is your body's most powerful recovery tool.

Morning Weigh-In

Each morning, weigh yourself the same way, at the same time, to stay consistent. Don't worry about daily fluctuations—watch for trends over time. As your glucose balance improves, your energy, sleep, and body composition will follow.

Glucose-Smart Habits

Before you eat:

- Drink a glass of water with a teaspoon of apple cider vinegar.

- Do a 5–10 minute "exercise snack" (light resistance moves or squats) to activate your muscles—they'll absorb glucose more efficiently at your next meal.

After you eat:

- Take a **10–15 minute walk** to help your glucose levels return to balance.

Date/Time	Before/ After	Eat/ Exercise	Meal/ Activity	Glucose

🙂 Glucose under 100 — you're in balance

☹️ Glucose above 100 — an opportunity to adjust

Chapter 17: Clinical Practice Guideline: Optimizing Body Composition During Weight Management

1.0 Introduction and Guideline Scope

1.1 The Clinical Challenge: Weight Loss and Muscle Mass Preservation

Weight loss is a cornerstone of therapy for managing obesity and its associated comorbidities. However, standard weight management interventions present a significant clinical challenge: the concurrent and unintentional loss of metabolically active skeletal muscle mass (SMM). Evidence demonstrates that during weight reduction, 20-40% of the total weight lost is typically derived from fat-free mass (FFM), which includes skeletal muscle. This loss is metabolically detrimental, as it can reduce resting metabolic rate, diminish physical capacity, and negatively impact long-term health and function.

Repeated cycles of weight loss and regain, or the natural aging process, can exacerbate this issue, leading to a condition known as sarcopenic obesity. This state is characterized by an unhealthy imbalance of excess fat mass and depleted skeletal muscle, which significantly increases the risk for metabolic disease. Therefore, the quality of weight lost—prioritizing fat mass over lean mass—is as critical as the quantity.

The primary objective of this guideline is to provide evidence-based, actionable recommendations for healthcare professionals. These recommendations are designed to help structure weight management interventions that maximize the loss of fat mass while strategically preserving SMM, thereby improving overall metabolic health and long-term patient outcomes.

1.2 Target Audience and Patient Population

This guideline is intended for healthcare professionals actively involved in weight management, including physicians, advanced practice practitioners, registered dietitians, physical therapists, pharmacists, and diabetes educators.

The target patient population includes adults with overweight or obesity, defined as a Body Mass Index (BMI) of ≥ 25 kg/m². Particular attention should be given to populations at higher risk for accelerated SMM loss during weight management. These include the elderly and post-menopausal women. Furthermore, evidence suggests ethnic differences can influence SMM loss; for example, in premenopausal women, those of European-American descent may lose more muscle with weight loss compared to African-American women when resistance exercise is not incorporated into the regimen. A thorough initial patient assessment is the crucial first step in developing a personalized and effective treatment plan.

2.0 Foundational Principles: Patient Assessment and Goal Setting

2.1 Comprehensive Initial Evaluation

A comprehensive initial patient assessment is a strategic imperative that forms the foundation of a personalized, safe, and effective weight management plan. This evaluation allows clinicians to look beyond simple weight reduction and focus on the more clinically relevant goal of optimizing body composition to improve metabolic health.

The initial assessment should include the following key components:

- **Metabolic Profile:** A baseline assessment of key metabolic health markers is essential. This includes measuring HbA1c, fasting blood glucose, and a complete lipid profile to evaluate glycemic control and dyslipidemia.

- **Body Composition:** Quantification of body composition beyond BMI is critical to establish a baseline for fat mass, FFM, and visceral adipose tissue (VAT). Recommended methods include dual-energy X-ray absorptiometry (DXA), bioelectrical impedance analysis (BIA), and waist circumference measurement as a surrogate marker for visceral adiposity.

- **Comorbidity Screening:** Patients should be screened for common obesity-related comorbidities, including dyslipidemia, hypertension, type 2 diabetes mellitus (T2DM), non-alcoholic fatty liver disease (NAFLD), obstructive sleep apnea, and osteoarthritis.

- **Identification of At-Risk Status:** The evaluation must identify patients at higher risk for disproportionate SMM loss during weight reduction. This includes, but is not limited to, older adults and post-menopausal women, who are particularly vulnerable to sarcopenia.

2.2 Establishing Holistic Treatment Goals

Effective treatment goals must extend beyond a target number on a scale. Evidence shows that significant metabolic improvements, such as prediabetes remission, can occur independently of weight loss and are more closely associated with healthier fat distribution. Therefore, goals should be holistic, incorporating improvements in body composition and metabolic markers.

- **Clinically Meaningful Weight Loss:** A target weight loss of 5-15% of initial body weight should be established as a primary goal. This range is clinically meaningful and sufficient to achieve significant improvements in cardiometabolic parameters, including blood pressure, lipids, and glycemic control.

- **Body Composition and Metabolic Markers:** In addition to weight, goals should include a reduction in waist circumference (reflecting a decrease in VAT) and improvements in the metabolic profile (e.g., lower HbA1c, improved lipid levels).

Achieving these goals requires a multi-faceted approach that integrates specific nutritional and exercise strategies designed to preferentially target fat mass while sparing lean tissue.

3.0 Core Recommendation 1: Nutritional Strategies for Muscle Sparing

3.1 The Critical Role of Dietary Protein

Dietary intervention is a fundamental component of any weight management program, but the macronutrient composition of the diet is critical for preserving metabolically active tissue. Among all macronutrients, dietary protein is the most important for mitigating the loss of FFM and SMM during periods of energy restriction. The standard Recommended Daily Allowance (RDA) for protein (0.8 g/kg body weight/day) may be insufficient to preserve lean mass during active weight loss, as studies have shown that inadequate protein intake during caloric restriction may be associated with adverse body-composition changes.

Evidence strongly supports a higher protein intake to create an anabolic stimulus that protects muscle tissue.

- **General Recommendation:** Protein intake during active weight loss should exceed **1.0 g/kg body weight/day.**

- **Optimal Target Range:** Clinical studies demonstrate that an intake of **1.2 g/kg to 1.6 g/kg of body weight/day** provides superior preservation of FFM compared to lower protein diets.

- **Special Populations:** Older individuals may derive the most significant benefit from higher protein intake to counteract age-related anabolic resistance and SMM loss.

Emphasis should also be placed on protein quality. High-quality protein sources, such as lean meat, fish, and whey protein, are rich in essential amino acids (particularly leucine) that are key for stimulating muscle protein synthesis.

3.2 Carbohydrate Modification and Overall Dietary Pattern

A carbohydrate-restricted dietary approach can be an effective strategy for improving glycemic control, particularly in patients with prediabetes or T2DM. Studies have shown this approach leads to significant improvements in A1C and fasting blood glucose levels.

An effective low-carbohydrate diet should include:

- **Recommended Foods:** A focus on non-starchy vegetables, fish, poultry, lean meat, eggs, olive oil, avocados, and nuts.

- **Foods to Limit:** A reduction in other dairy products, fruits, legumes, beans, and grains.

Ultimately, long-term adherence is paramount for sustained success. The dietary plan must be sustainable for the individual. An approach centered on a healthy, "normocaloric" dietary pattern—one that focuses on diet quality rather than severe calorie restriction alone—can help patients implement durable lifestyle changes. This strategy, when combined with physical activity, forms a powerful and sustainable intervention.

4.0 Core Recommendation 2: Exercise Prescription for Optimizing Body Composition

4.1 The Synergy of Resistance and Aerobic Training

Exercise is a non-negotiable component of any weight management plan designed to optimize body composition. While dietary restriction drives weight loss, exercise dictates the quality of that loss. Resistance training and aerobic exercise play distinct yet synergistic roles. Resistance training is the most effective behavioral strategy for stimulating SMM growth and preservation, while aerobic exercise is highly effective at promoting fat loss and attenuating SMM loss during energy restriction.

Clinical evidence confirms that combining exercise with dietary modification significantly reduces FFM loss compared to diet alone. Therefore, a program that strategically integrates both resistance and aerobic training is superior for improving body composition.

4.2 Evidence-Based Resistance Training Protocols

A meta-analysis of resistance training in women provides specific, actionable protocols for maximizing strength gains, which are correlated with muscle preservation and growth. The optimal protocol differs for the upper and lower body, likely due to differences in muscle fiber distribution and typical patterns of use in daily life.

- **Lower-Body Training:**
    - **Intensity/Load:** Recommend training with heavy loads for 1 to 6 repetitions per set to maximize strength gains.

    - **Frequency:** Recommend training two times per week.

- **Upper-Body Training:**
    - **Intensity/Load:** Recommend training with lighter loads for 13 to 20 repetitions per set.

    - **Frequency:** Recommend training two to three times per week.

4.3 Role of Aerobic Exercise

Aerobic exercise is a critical tool for promoting fat loss and creating the necessary energy deficit for weight reduction, while also helping to attenuate the loss of SMM that can occur with energy restriction alone.

A moderate-intensity aerobic exercise regimen, such as **walking 3-5 times per week for 35-45 minutes**, is an effective and accessible example.

In summary, exercise, and particularly resistance training, is the most powerful behavioral strategy for directing weight loss toward the fat mass compartment. For appropriately selected patients, the benefits of lifestyle modification can be further enhanced by adjunctive pharmacotherapy.

5.0 Core Recommendation 3: Adjunctive Pharmacotherapy with GLP-1 Receptor Agonists

5.1 Role and Mechanism of Action

For appropriately selected patients, Glucagon-like Peptide-1 Receptor Agonists (GLP-1 RAs) are an effective **adjunct** to diet and exercise. Pharmacotherapy should never be considered a substitute for foundational lifestyle modification but rather a tool to enhance its effects.

The primary mechanisms by which GLP-1 RAs promote weight loss are centrally and peripherally mediated:

- **Reduced appetite and hunger** by acting on hypothalamic centers.

- **Increased satiety** (feelings of fullness).

- **Slowed gastric emptying**, which prolongs the feeling of fullness after a meal.

Emerging evidence also suggests that GLP-1 RAs may have direct beneficial effects on the musculoskeletal system. These pleiotropic effects include **inhibiting muscle atrophy, preserving muscle strength, and enhancing exercise endurance**, making them a compelling option in a muscle-sparing weight loss strategy.

5.2 Agent Selection and Clinical Considerations

Several GLP-1 RAs and dual-agonist therapies have demonstrated robust efficacy for weight management in clinical trials.

Agent	Class	Noted Efficacy in Clinical Trials for Weight Loss
Liraglutide	GLP-1 RA	An earlier-approved agent for chronic weight management.
Semaglutide	GLP-1 RA	Clinical trials demonstrated a greater average weight loss compared to liraglutide.
Tirzepatide	Dual GIP/GLP-1 RA	Demonstrated superior dose-dependent weight loss compared to semaglutide, with up to a 20.9% body weight reduction in the SURMOUNT-1 trial.

Patient Selection and Contraindications

- **Indications:** Pharmacotherapy should be considered for individuals with a BMI ≥30 kg/m² or a BMI ≥27 kg/m² with at least one weight-related comorbidity (e.g., T2DM, hypertension, dyslipidemia).

- **Contraindications and Cautions:**
    - GLP-1 RAs are contraindicated in patients with a personal or family history of medullary thyroid carcinoma (MTC) or Multiple Endocrine Neoplasia syndrome type 2 (MEN2).

    - They are also contraindicated in patients with a history of pancreatitis.

    - Agents should be avoided in patients with a history of gastroparesis or severe inflammatory bowel disorders.

    - Recent evidence has highlighted a higher risk of pancreatitis, gastroparesis, and bowel obstruction associated with GLP-1 agonist use for weight loss compared to other anti-obesity agents.

- **Common Adverse Effects:** The most common side effects are gastrointestinal in nature (nausea, vomiting, diarrhea). These effects are typically mild-to-moderate and tend to occur during the dose-escalation period.

Obesity is a chronic disease, and to prevent weight regain upon cessation, treatment with anti-obesity medications should be considered a long-term therapy. Success requires ongoing monitoring and support from an integrated care team.

6.0 Integrated Care and Long-Term Monitoring

6.1 The Interprofessional Team Approach

Optimizing long-term weight management outcomes and preserving metabolic health requires a coordinated, interprofessional team approach. A patient-centered, holistic team can provide comprehensive support, manage comorbidities, and enhance adherence. The ideal team includes:

- **Primary Care Physician/Advanced Practice Practitioner:** Manages overall health and coordinates care.

- **Endocrinologist:** Provides specialized care for complex metabolic disease and guides pharmacotherapy decisions.

- **Registered Dietitian:** Designs and guides personalized medical nutrition therapy to achieve protein targets and overall dietary goals.

- **Physical Therapist:** Develops safe and effective exercise prescriptions, ensuring proper form and progression, particularly for resistance training.

- **Pharmacist:** Educates on medication administration, manages side effects, and addresses cost/access issues.

- **Diabetes Educator/Nursing Staff:** Provides ongoing patient education, self-management support, and routine monitoring.

6.2 Key Monitoring Parameters

Long-term success depends on routine follow-up and monitoring of key parameters to track progress, ensure safety, and adjust the treatment plan as needed.

- **Body Composition:** Continue to monitor total body weight and waist circumference to track changes in overall mass and central adiposity.

- **Metabolic Health:** Regularly assess metabolic markers, including blood glucose levels, HbA1c, and lipid profiles, to ensure treatment goals are being met and maintained.

- **Kidney Function:** Monitor renal function (e.g., eGFR, UACR) as part of routine laboratory follow-up.

- **Hematologic Parameters:** Monitor a complete blood count (CBC) as indicated.

- **Treatment Adherence and Tolerability:** Conduct routine follow-ups to assess adherence to diet and exercise plans. For patients on pharmacotherapy, monitor for and manage any adverse effects to ensure tolerability and continued use.

A successful weight management strategy is one that is sustainable and prioritizes the quality of weight lost. By focusing on maximizing fat loss while preserving skeletal muscle, clinicians can help patients achieve not just a lower number on the scale, but a profound and lasting improvement in overall metabolic health.

The Independent Contribution of Physical Activity

Lifestyle factors, particularly physical activity, play an independent and significant role in modulating insulin sensitivity.

- **Vigorous Activity is Key:** The study by Clamp et al. found that vigorous physical activity was a significant predictor of improved insulin sensitivity.

- **Reducing Sedentary Time:** Increasing light activity at the expense of sedentary time was also shown to improve fasting measures of insulin sensitivity (HOMA-IR).

- **Quantifiable Impact:** Regression modeling from the study demonstrated that a predicted 15% improvement in HOMA-IR could be achieved through an additional 55 minutes of light activity or just 5 minutes of vigorous activity per day. This highlights the potency of high-intensity exercise.

- **Independence from Diet:** In the Clamp et al. study, physical activity variables were significant predictors of insulin sensitivity, whereas dietary intake variables were not, emphasizing the unique and powerful role of exercise.

Whew! — that was a lot of science!!

And yet, this is the beauty of it all: the science simply proves what women have always known deep down — that our bodies are powerful, adaptable, and wise when we finally listen to them.

You've just read the research, the numbers, the data — but the real transformation happens in the quiet moments when you apply it. When you nourish instead of deprive. When you lift with strength instead of fear. When you choose rest as an act of progress, not weakness.

Reinvented isn't just a framework; it's a conversation — between your biology and your belief in what's possible. It's a return to harmony, to confidence, to energy that lasts.
So as you close this book, remember: you are not starting over. You are starting **in alignment** — with knowledge, intention, and grace.

Science gave us the blueprint.
You bring it to life.

Here's to strength that shows, energy that radiates, and health that feels like freedom.

Chapter 18:
Recap of The Reinvented Framework: Your Metabolic Blueprint

Your body isn't the problem — it's the guide. Reinvented helps you learn its language.

This framework was designed to help you balance hormones, stabilize energy, and reshape body composition by focusing on what truly drives health at every stage of life. It's not a diet or a temporary fix. It's a system built on four pillars: **Fuel, Move, Recover, and Track.**

Think of it as your personal blueprint — one that adapts to you, your season of life, and your goals. The Reinvented Framework isn't about restriction or willpower. It's about rhythm, awareness, and alignment with your biology.

PILLAR 1: FUEL — Nourish, Don't Punish

Goal: Stabilize glucose, protect muscle, and nourish your hormones.

Food is not the enemy — it's information. Every meal sends a message to your body about whether to store fat or burn it, build muscle or break it down. Reinvented teaches you to use food strategically to create balance and metabolic calm.

Core Principles:

- **Prioritize Protein:** Aim for 1.2–1.6g per kilogram (or 0.55–0.75g per pound) of body weight daily. Protein is the foundation for muscle, hormone synthesis, and satiety.

- **Pair Smartly:** Combine carbs with protein, fiber, or fat to blunt glucose spikes and keep energy stable.

- **Eat Mindfully:** Slow down. Chew well. Stop when 80% full. This isn't deprivation — it's discernment.

- **Time with Intention:** If meals are spaced more than 4 hours apart, have a protein-rich snack. Skipping meals may work for men, but for most women, it raises cortisol and disrupts glucose balance.

- Hydrate + Mineralize: Add electrolytes, especially magnesium and potassium, to support metabolism and prevent fatigue.

Glucose-Friendly Meal Framework:

- **Morning:** Protein + fiber → Steady energy, balanced cortisol.

- **Midday:** Protein + complex carbs → Support focus and muscle synthesis.

- **Evening:** Protein + veggies + healthy fats → Satiety without glucose overload.

Remember: Food isn't about control — it's about communication. Each choice is a message of support, not punishment.

PILLAR 2: MOVE — Build Strength, Build Stability

Goal: Use movement to reshape your metabolism, not just your body.

Exercise determines what kind of weight you lose — and keep. When you build and protect muscle, you preserve your metabolic engine.

The Reinvented Movement Formula:

- **3x Strength Training:** Resistance exercises targeting all major muscle groups. Prioritize progressive overload (gradually increasing resistance).

- **2x Aerobic Training:** Brisk walks, cycling, swimming — Zone 2 cardio to improve fat metabolism and endurance.

- **2x Mobility & Flexibility:** Pilates, yoga, or stretching to maintain joint health and balance cortisol.

- **Daily Activity:** Move often. 10-minute walks after meals reduce glucose spikes and enhance digestion.

Key Truths:

- Muscle is metabolic gold — every pound burns glucose and fat 24/7.

- Cardio trims fat, but strength training transforms your shape.

- Flexibility keeps you moving — literally and hormonally.

Example Weekly Blueprint:

- **Mon:** Lower-body strength
- **Tue:** HIIT or Zone 2 cardio
- **Wed:** Upper-body strength
- **Thu:** Pilates or yoga
- **Fri:** Full-body strength
- **Sat:** Active fun (hike, dance, bike, play)
- **Sun:** Rest + mobility

The goal is consistency, not perfection. Your body doesn't need punishment — it needs participation.

PILLAR 3: RECOVER — Rest is the Real Work

Goal: Restore balance through sleep, stress regulation, and emotional recovery.

Cortisol, your stress hormone, has a direct relationship with glucose. When stress stays high, insulin resistance increases — and fat storage follows.
Recovery is the secret weapon in body transformation because it restores your hormones, nervous system, and energy capacity.

Daily Recovery Rituals:

- **Sleep Hygiene:** Aim for 7–9 hours. Keep the room cool, dark, and quiet. Avoid screens 1 hour before bed.

- **Evening Reset:** Journal, stretch, or practice breathwork to downshift your nervous system.

- **Stress Management:** Schedule pauses. Walks, baths, nature, laughter, music — they all count as medicine.

- **Rest Days = Growth Days:** Muscle rebuilds during rest, not during training.

Sleep, Cortisol, and Glucose:

Even one night of poor sleep can elevate glucose the next day and trigger cravings. Treat sleep like nutrition — it fuels everything else.

PILLAR 4: TRACK — Data with Compassion

Goal: Use awareness as your most powerful tool.

Self-tracking transforms abstract advice into actionable insight. It's not about numbers; it's about *noticing*.

How to Track:

- **Withings Scale:** Weekly check-ins for muscle and fat composition.

- **RENPHO Tape:** Measure waist-to-hip ratio biweekly for progress.

- **WHOOP Band:** Monitor sleep, recovery, and heart rate variability.

- **CGM or Glucose Monitor:** Observe your body's real-time responses to food, movement, and stress.

- **Journal:** Note energy, mood, and digestion — the qualitative side of the data.

Reflection Prompts for Tracking:

1. When did I feel most balanced this week?

2. What foods or habits supported my energy best?

3. Where did I feel resistance — and what might it be teaching me?

Tracking isn't about control; it's about connection. When you track with curiosity, you reclaim authorship of your own story.

The Reinvented Rhythm

When all four pillars — Fuel, Move, Recover, Track — work together, your body finds balance naturally.

You:
- Build muscle, not just burn calories.

- Steady energy, not chase caffeine.

- Sleep deeper, stress less, glow more.

This is the reinvention: from reactive to responsive, from guessing to guided, from striving to *thriving*.

The Reinvented Framework is your daily practice of becoming — not someone new, but more wholly *you*.

How to Live Reinvented: The 7 Daily Practices

A guide to living in rhythm with your biology, not against it.

You don't need a perfect plan to feel balanced — you need rhythm.

These seven daily practices are the heartbeat of the *Reinvented* lifestyle — small, intentional actions that align your hormones, metabolism, and energy with the natural flow of the day.

When you live in tune with your body, every day becomes a practice in health, not a test of willpower.

1. Wake with Light

"The first light you see should come from the sun, not your screen."

Morning sunlight is one of the simplest, most powerful metabolic resets available.
Within 10–15 minutes of waking, step outside — no sunglasses, no phone.
Natural light activates photoreceptors in your eyes that regulate cortisol and melatonin, helping you wake up naturally, stabilize mood, and improve sleep quality later.

Science shows that morning light helps synchronize your circadian rhythm — the internal clock that governs hormones, hunger, and metabolism. Women who align their routines with natural light experience better insulin sensitivity and energy throughout the day.

Try this:

While you sip your coffee or tea, take a short walk, stretch, or simply breathe. This is your first act of self-regulation — and the day's first signal to your body that you're safe, awake, and in rhythm.

2. Move Before You Scroll

Before the digital noise begins, give your body a chance to lead. Just five minutes of gentle movement — stretching, walking, light strength work, or Pilates — wakes up your lymphatic system, increases circulation, and lowers cortisol spikes that often happen from morning stress or scrolling.

If you strength train later in the day, this gentle morning movement still sets the tone for metabolic flexibility. It signals your muscles to engage glucose more efficiently — a quiet biochemical upgrade that happens before your inbox even opens.

Try this:

Keep a yoga mat or resistance band near your bedside. Before you reach for your phone, do five slow squats, five pushups against the wall, or one minute of deep breathing with your arms overhead. One small act of movement creates momentum for the rest of the day.

3. Eat with Presence

How you eat matters as much as what you eat.

When you rush through meals, your nervous system remains in "fight or flight" mode, impairing digestion and spiking glucose. Slowing down before eating helps your body shift into "rest and digest," the parasympathetic state that supports stable blood sugar and nutrient absorption.

Try this:

Before you take your first bite, pause. Take three deep breaths. Look at your food — the colors, the textures, the care that went into it.
This small ritual of awareness can reduce post-meal glucose spikes by as much as 20–30% according to emerging studies on mindfulness and metabolism.

Presence transforms eating from an unconscious act into a metabolic meditation.

4. Strength Before Cardio

When you move, move with intention.

Most women are taught to "burn calories" — but what truly reshapes your metabolism is building muscle. Strength training first, before long cardio, primes your body to use glucose efficiently and protects lean tissue.

Muscle is more than aesthetic — it's hormonal. It acts as an endocrine organ, releasing myokines that improve insulin sensitivity and reduce inflammation.

When you lift weights, you're not just training your body — you're recalibrating your biology.

Try this:
Lift 2–3 times per week. Prioritize form over intensity, consistency over duration.

If time is short, focus on compound moves — squats, lunges, pushups, and rows.

Each rep is a message to your metabolism that strength is the goal, not depletion.

5. Recover Like You Train

Rest isn't a reward — it's a requirement.

Every rep, every walk, every deep breath you take adds to your recovery account. Yet most women overdraw that account daily.

When you train hard but sleep little, when you give endlessly but pause rarely, you signal to your body that survival is more important than repair.

Try this:

- Build "recovery appointments" into your calendar: a bath, a nap, a walk without purpose.

- Treat rest like a workout — with structure and intention.

- Embrace silence. Physiological recovery starts when mental noise stops.

Your metabolism is shaped as much by recovery as by training.

6. Reflect + Track

Self-awareness is data in motion.

Tracking doesn't have to be obsessive — it can be compassionate. The goal isn't perfection, but pattern recognition.

Use your **Withings scale** weekly to monitor fat vs. muscle.
Use the **RENPHO tape** biweekly to track waist and hip changes.
Use your **WHOOP band** or smartwatch to notice recovery trends.
If you use a glucose monitor, treat it as feedback, not judgment.

Then, record what really matters: how you feel.
When were you most calm? Most strong? Most alive?

This is how numbers become narrative — and narrative becomes transformation.

7. Sleep to Transform

If you do nothing else, protect your sleep.

Sleep is when your body repairs muscle, balances hormones, and consolidates memory — the true recovery zone. Yet for many women, midlife sleep disruption is one of the first and most frustrating symptoms of hormonal change.

The good news? You can restore your rhythm.

Try this:

- Keep bedtime consistent — aim for 7–9 hours nightly.

- Dim lights 90 minutes before sleep; avoid screens or use blue-light filters.

- Consider supplements like magnesium glycinate or L-theanine for relaxation.

- Treat your bedroom like a sanctuary: cool, dark, and uncluttered.

Sleep isn't passive — it's the most productive thing you'll do for your metabolism all day.

The Art of Consistency

Living *Reinvented* isn't about rigid rules — it's about alignment. When you follow these seven practices with kindness and consistency, your biology responds with balance.
Your energy evens out. Your hunger stabilizes. Your body composition shifts naturally toward strength and equilibrium.

You don't have to overhaul your life overnight.
Start with one ritual, one rhythm, one moment of presence.

Because becoming *Reinvented* doesn't happen in a day — it happens every day.
Quietly. Gracefully. In the small choices that whisper:
"I'm ready to work with my body, not against it."

Chapter 19:
The Science of Longevity for Women

Because living better is how you live longer.

Longevity has become the new language of wellness, but for women, it's more than extending years — it's extending quality. The goal is not just to live longer, but to stay vibrant, mobile, strong, and sharp through every decade.

Modern science now shows that the foundation of female longevity isn't mystery — it's muscle, metabolism, and mindset. Each plays a crucial role in how gracefully we age and how well we continue to feel at home in our bodies.

1. Muscle: The True Marker of Youth

Forget what you've been told — the real anti-aging secret isn't found in a jar or a pill. It's found in your muscles.

Muscle is the most underrated organ of longevity. Beyond strength and tone, it's an active endocrine system — constantly communicating with your metabolism, your brain, and even your immune cells. It releases molecules called **myokines** that reduce inflammation, improve insulin sensitivity, and protect cognitive function.

Studies show that women with higher muscle mass have significantly lower risks of metabolic syndrome, osteoporosis, dementia, and premature mortality. In fact, muscle mass and grip strength are now used as clinical predictors of lifespan.

The takeaway:
If you want to age beautifully, train for strength.
Lift weights. Carry groceries. Garden. Walk up the stairs.
Every act of resistance builds resilience.

When you build muscle, you're not only shaping your body — you're securing your future.

2. Metabolism: The Energy of Youth

Most people think metabolism "slows down" with age — but that's not entirely true. What changes is the efficiency of energy use, largely driven by hormone shifts, muscle loss, and stress load.

When estrogen begins to decline, glucose regulation becomes more difficult. Cortisol rises more easily. Sleep becomes lighter, and cravings louder. But this isn't a breakdown — it's a recalibration.

Your metabolism is a communication system between food, muscle, and hormones. When you balance glucose, nourish with protein, and manage stress, you re-educate that system. It begins to work *with* you again.

Metabolic health is longevity health. It determines how well your brain functions, how stable your mood feels, and how efficiently your cells repair themselves.

Simple longevity upgrades:

- Eat 30–40g of protein per meal.

- Move daily (especially resistance + walking).

- Sleep deeply.

- Keep glucose steady — not perfect, just stable.

- Fast only if it supports your energy, not drains it.

Metabolism isn't lost — it's learned.

3. Mitochondria: Your Cellular Power Source

At the most microscopic level, longevity lives in your **mitochondria** — the powerhouses of every cell. These tiny engines convert food into usable energy. When they're healthy, you feel it: clear mind, steady energy, glowing skin, and emotional balance.

As we age, mitochondrial efficiency declines — but it's not inevitable. The same practices that balance glucose and strengthen muscle also reignite these cellular engines.

Mitochondrial boosters include:

- Resistance training (stimulates new mitochondria growth).

- Cold exposure or contrast showers (activates fat metabolism).
- Nutrients like CoQ10, omega-3s, and magnesium.

- Quality sleep and sunlight exposure.

When you train your body, you train your cells. And when your cells thrive, aging slows.

4. Hormones: The Symphony of Adaptation

Hormones are not just chemical messengers — they're conductors of your entire internal orchestra. Estrogen, progesterone, thyroid, and cortisol all dance together, influencing how you burn energy, store fat, and recover.

The *Reinvented* framework treats hormonal changes not as a crisis, but as communication.
Perimenopause and menopause are not endings — they're transitions.
When supported through nourishment, movement, and mindfulness, they can become the most grounded, confident, and vibrant years of your life.

Hormonal balance = metabolic grace.

5. Brain Health: The Overlooked Frontier

One of the most profound insights in longevity science is the connection between **muscle and mind.**

Regular resistance and aerobic exercise stimulate **BDNF (brain-derived neurotrophic factor)** — a growth factor that supports memory, mood, and cognitive clarity.

Women who train regularly have a 30–40% lower risk of cognitive decline.
And even beyond the data, movement lifts more than weights — it lifts fog, fear, and fatigue.

Your brain craves movement as much as your muscles do.

6. Emotional Longevity: Joy, Purpose, and Connection

There's another form of aging science can't quite measure — the energy of joy.
Oxytocin, serotonin, and dopamine — the "feel-good" hormones — are potent longevity molecules. They're released when you laugh, connect, create, or give.

Longevity researchers consistently find that **social connection** is one of the strongest predictors of lifespan — especially in women. When we gather, share, and support one another, we literally extend each other's vitality.

That's why *Reinvented* isn't just a book — it's a movement. It's community medicine.

Every shared meal, walk, or conversation between women is a dose of anti-aging chemistry — and the most natural therapy on earth.

7. The Longevity Loop: Integration Over Perfection

Longevity is not achieved through extremes — it's earned through consistency.
You don't need to be perfect. You need to be *present*.

The habits that keep you young are the same ones that keep you grounded:

- Eat real food, not empty calories.

- Move daily, not endlessly.

- Rest deeply, not guiltily.

- Connect authentically, not performatively.

If you do these simple things most of the time, your biology thanks you all of the time.

8. The Reinvented Longevity Formula

To age well as a woman is to rewrite the script society handed us.
It's to replace decline with discovery.
To trade fear of change for mastery of evolution.

The Reinvented Longevity Formula is beautifully simple:

> **Strong Muscle + Stable Glucose + Rested Mind = Ageless Energy**

Longevity isn't about stopping time — it's about aligning with it.

When your body, hormones, and energy move in harmony, aging stops being something that happens to you and becomes something that happens *with you.*

You don't fight it — you flow with it.
You don't resist it — you reinvent it.

Because the future of wellness isn't found in youth — it's found in vitality.
And the most radiant women aren't the youngest — they're the most aligned.

Longevity isn't measured in years lived, but in energy expressed.

When you wake with purpose, move with strength, eat with intention, and rest with reverence — every decade becomes your best one yet.

Epilogue: The Science of Becoming

You've made it to the end — but really, this is the beginning.

Somewhere between the data, the workouts, the meals, and the mindfulness, something shifted. You stopped trying to *fix* your body — and started listening to it. You began to see your metabolism not as an enemy, but as a messenger. You started to understand that health isn't something to chase — it's something to *allow*.

We live in a culture that glorifies effort but undervalues ease. We measure worth in steps, macros, and deadlines — forgetting that the deepest healing often happens in the quiet. Reinvented is an invitation to remember that your biology is not broken. It's brilliant. It's adaptive. It's been waiting for you to stop fighting and start flowing with it.

You've learned how glucose fuels energy, how muscle guards longevity, how sleep and stress sculpt your hormones. But beneath the science lies something more sacred — self-trust. The quiet knowing that you are capable of caring for yourself with both intelligence and grace.

Because the truth is: transformation isn't about *discipline*. It's about *devotion*.
Devotion to your body.
Devotion to your energy.
Devotion to your becoming.

The woman who began this journey may have been tired, frustrated, or doubting her reflection. But the woman reading these words now — she knows better. She knows that her body is not the past she must correct, but the future she can create.

You are not here to return to who you were.
You are here to rise into who you've always been.

So take what you've learned — the science, the structure, the stillness — and live it.
Walk slower. Lift stronger. Eat with intention. Rest with reverence.
Let every small, consistent act become a quiet declaration of your new identity:

You are not a project. You are a masterpiece in motion. You are not chasing youth. You are cultivating longevity. You are not waiting to be chosen. You are choosing yourself.

Your body has never stopped communicating with you.
Now, finally, you're fluent.

You are — and always have been — *Reinvented*.

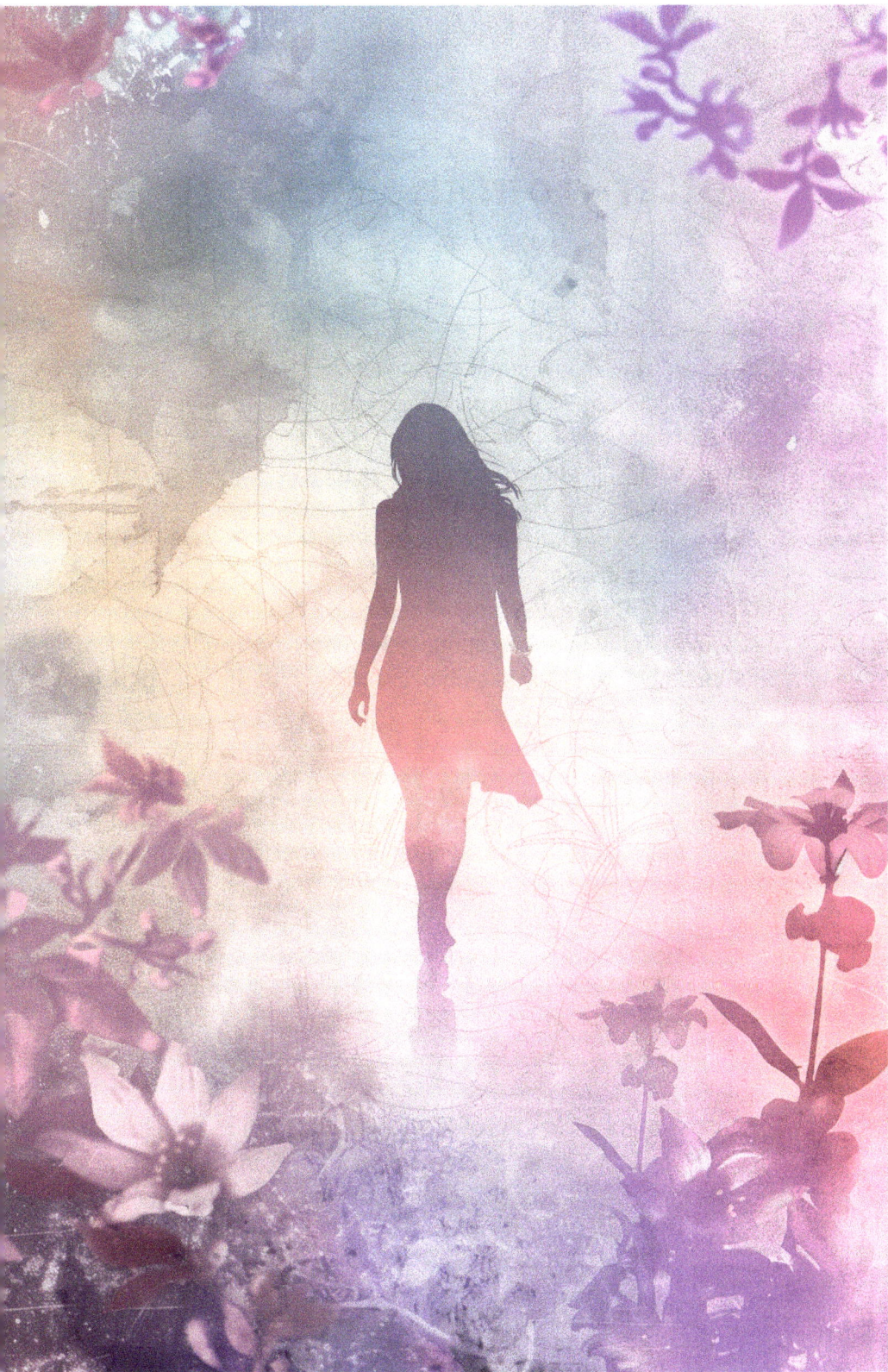

Letter from the Authors

Dear Reader,

You've just completed a journey through *Reinvented*—a framework designed for women ready to reclaim control of their bodies, energy, and confidence. This book isn't just about information; it's the result of decades of research, coaching, and lived experience. It's about redefining what's possible for women at every stage of life.

Cho Phillips created *The Glucose Blueprint Framework* after years of research and science-backed studies focused specifically on women. She tested and refined these principles in her own life—and in the lives of countless women—who had struggled for years before finally seeing extraordinary results through this approach.

Debra Hohmann, MSN, APRN, FNP-BC, brings her expertise in obesity medicine, hormone health, and preventive care to the heart of this book. As a board-certified nurse practitioner, Debra has spent her career helping women navigate the complex changes of midlife with compassion and evidence-based guidance. Her mission is to help women understand their bodies, balance their hormones, and move through this next phase of life with clarity, confidence, and vitality. To her, menopause care isn't about symptom management—it's about empowerment.

Brooke Preston, Plant-Based Whole Food Nutrition and Holistic Health Coach, curated the *Nutritional Meal Plans and Recipes* designed to fuel your body, balance your hormones, and stabilize glucose—while bringing joy back to eating well.

Together, we've built a blueprint that's simple, sustainable, and deeply personal. It's not about restriction—it's about *reinvention*.

We know this works because we've lived it, coached it, and witnessed it. We've seen women who once felt "broken" by their hormones or stuck in endless dieting cycles unlock results they never thought possible: fat loss, muscle gain, steady energy, and renewed self-trust.

Now it's your turn. This is your invitation to stop chasing diets and start creating a lifestyle that works with your body—not against it. Your blueprint won't look like anyone else's, and that's the point. It's uniquely yours.

We're honored to guide you on this journey—and we can't wait to see the woman you become.

With strength, health, and unstoppable confidence,
Cho, Debra, and Brooke

Join The Reinvented Collective

A private coaching community for women redefining strength, balance, and longevity.

Transformation doesn't happen in isolation — it happens in connection.

If you've read *Reinvented* and felt inspired to take action but know you'd benefit from more guidance, accountability, or encouragement, we created something just for you.

The Reinvented Collective is our private coaching community for women ready to turn knowledge into results.

Inside, you'll find:

- **Science-backed coaching** to help you navigate hormones, metabolism, and mindset with confidence.

- **Practical support** for nutrition, workouts, and lifestyle changes that actually last.

- **Community encouragement** from women on the same journey toward renewed energy, strength, and self-trust.

This is where information becomes transformation — and where you learn to build consistency, compassion, and confidence one step at a time.

Because reinvention isn't just about what you do — it's about who you become.

Join *The Reinvented Collective* on Facebook and connect with a community designed to help you create your healthiest, happiest chapter yet.

- facebook.com/groups/Reinvented

Glossary of Terms

A guide to the language of your body — and your reinvention.

A

Aging, Biological
The natural process of cellular and metabolic slowdown over time. Unlike chronological age (the number of birthdays you've had), biological age reflects how well your body is functioning.

Amino Acids
The building blocks of protein. Essential for repairing tissue, building muscle, and supporting hormones, enzymes, and neurotransmitters.

Anabolic State
A phase when your body is building up — creating new muscle, tissue, and energy stores. Often supported by adequate protein, sleep, and resistance training.

B

Basal Metabolic Rate (BMR)
The number of calories your body burns at rest to maintain vital functions like breathing, circulation, and cellular repair.

Biofeedback
Real-time signals from your body — such as heart rate, glucose, or energy levels — that reflect how it's responding to your environment, food, or stress.

Body Composition
The ratio of fat, muscle, bone, and water that make up your total body weight. A more accurate reflection of health than the scale alone.

Blood Glucose (Blood Sugar)
The amount of sugar (glucose) circulating in your bloodstream at a given moment. It fuels your body but can be harmful when chronically high.

C

Cortisol
A stress hormone released by the adrenal glands. In short bursts, it helps you wake up and stay alert; in chronic excess, it contributes to belly fat, fatigue, and poor sleep.

Creatine
A naturally occurring compound stored in muscles that provides quick energy during strength training. Supplementation can enhance muscle growth and recovery.

Continuous Glucose Monitor (CGM)
A wearable device that tracks glucose levels throughout the day and night, offering insights into how meals, sleep, and movement affect metabolism.

D

DEXA Scan
(Dual-Energy X-Ray Absorptiometry) — a medical test that measures bone density and body composition, providing a detailed look at fat and muscle distribution.

Dysregulation
When a system in the body — like glucose control or hormone balance — becomes unstable or inefficient, often due to stress, poor sleep, or diet.

E

Estrogen
A key female hormone that regulates menstrual cycles, metabolism, and fat storage. Its decline during perimenopause and menopause contributes to body composition changes.

Energy Availability
The amount of energy left for your body's essential functions after accounting for exercise. Low energy availability can disrupt hormones and slow metabolism.

F

Fat-Free Mass (FFM)
Everything in your body that isn't fat — including muscle, bone, water, and organs.

Functional Training
Exercise that mimics everyday movement — such as squats, lunges, or lifts — improving strength, coordination, and balance.

G

Glucose
Your body's main source of fuel, derived from carbohydrates. Balanced glucose supports steady energy, mood, and fat metabolism.

GLP-1 (Glucagon-Like Peptide-1)
A hormone that promotes satiety and regulates blood sugar. Certain medications (GLP-1 receptor agonists) mimic its effects for weight management.

Glycogen
Stored glucose found in muscles and the liver, used for quick energy during activity or fasting.

H

Heart Rate Variability (HRV)
A measure of the variation between heartbeats — a marker of nervous system balance and recovery. Higher HRV generally reflects better stress resilience.

Hormone Replacement Therapy (HRT)
Medical treatment that supplements estrogen and/or progesterone levels to relieve menopausal symptoms and support bone and metabolic health.

Homeostasis
Your body's natural tendency to maintain internal balance — temperature, pH, glucose, and more.

I

Insulin
A hormone that helps move glucose from the bloodstream into cells for energy. Chronic excess insulin can lead to insulin resistance.

Insulin Resistance
When cells become less responsive to insulin, causing glucose to stay elevated in the blood. Common during midlife and menopause, but reversible through lifestyle changes.

Inflammation

The body's natural response to stress or injury. Chronic, low-grade inflammation is linked to aging and metabolic disorders.

J

Journal Tracking

A mindful habit of recording meals, workouts, mood, and sleep to identify patterns and progress. Part data, part reflection, all self-awareness.

K

Ketones

Energy molecules produced when the body burns fat instead of glucose for fuel, often during fasting or low-carb diets.

K2 (Vitamin K2)

A fat-soluble vitamin that helps direct calcium to bones and away from arteries, supporting bone and cardiovascular health.

L

Lean Mass

The weight of everything in your body that isn't fat — primarily muscle, bones, and organs.

Leptin

A hormone produced by fat cells that signals fullness and helps regulate appetite. Leptin resistance can make it harder to feel satisfied after eating.

Longevity

Not just the length of life, but the quality of it — healthspan over lifespan.

M

Macronutrients (Macros)

The three main nutrient categories — protein, carbohydrates, and fat — that provide energy and structure for the body.

Magnesium

A mineral crucial for over 300 enzymatic processes, including sleep quality, glucose metabolism, and stress regulation.

Metabolic Flexibility

The body's ability to switch efficiently between burning carbs and fat for fuel. A key goal of glucose control.

Menopause

The natural end of menstrual cycles, marked by 12 months without a period. Often accompanied by hormonal shifts affecting metabolism and energy.

N

Nutrient Timing
Planning when you eat — especially protein and carbs — to optimize energy, recovery, and glucose balance.

Neuroplasticity
The brain's ability to adapt, grow, and rewire itself throughout life. Exercise, sleep, and mindfulness enhance it.

O

Omega-3 Fatty Acids
Essential fats that reduce inflammation and support brain, heart, and joint health. Found in fish, flaxseeds, and walnuts.

Oxidative Stress
A process caused by free radicals that can damage cells over time. Antioxidant-rich foods help counteract it.

P

Perimenopause
The transitional phase leading up to menopause, often marked by hormonal fluctuations, changes in cycle regularity, and shifts in mood, sleep, and metabolism.

Progressive Overload
Gradually increasing resistance or intensity in workouts to continue building strength and muscle.

Protein Quality
A measure of how well a protein source provides essential amino acids. Animal proteins and certain plant combinations offer the best profiles.

R

Recovery
The period after exercise when your body rebuilds muscle, restores energy, and adapts. As important as the workout itself.

Resting Metabolic Rate (RMR)
The amount of energy your body uses at rest — influenced by muscle mass, hormones, and age.

S

Sarcopenia
The natural loss of muscle mass and strength that occurs with aging — accelerated by inactivity but reversible with resistance training and proper nutrition.

Satiety
The feeling of fullness and satisfaction after eating, influenced by hormones like GLP-1, leptin, and ghrelin.

Sleep Hygiene
Habits and environment that support restful sleep — such as consistent bedtimes, reduced blue light, and calming routines.

T

Thermogenesis
The production of heat in the body. Certain foods (like protein) and activities (like resistance training) increase thermogenesis and calorie burn.

Thyroid Hormone
Regulates metabolism, energy, and temperature. Imbalances can cause fatigue, weight changes, and mood shifts.

Tracking (Self-Tracking)
The practice of observing measurable behaviors — like glucose, steps, or sleep — to improve self-awareness and habits.

V

Visceral Fat
Fat stored around internal organs in the abdomen. More metabolically active (and riskier) than subcutaneous fat but responsive to glucose control and exercise.

Vitamin D
Supports bone health, immune function, and mood regulation. Works synergistically with vitamin K2.

W

Weight Training (Resistance Training)
Using resistance (weights, bands, or body weight) to strengthen muscles, bones, and metabolism.

Withings Scale
A smart scale that measures body composition metrics like fat and muscle mass — used throughout Reinvented for tracking real progress.

WHOOP Band
A wearable device that measures recovery, strain, and sleep — helping you balance training intensity with rest.

Z

Zone 2 Training
Low-to-moderate intensity exercise (like brisk walking) that improves endurance and fat metabolism while lowering glucose levels.

Disclaimer Reminder

This book is intended for educational purposes only and should not be considered medical advice. Readers should consult with a qualified healthcare professional before beginning any new health, diet, or exercise program. Neither the publisher nor the authors assume any responsibility for the use or misuse of the information contained herein.

Your hormones aren't broken. Your blueprint just needs an update.

For too long, women in midlife have been told that weight gain, fatigue, and muscle loss are "just part of aging." But new research tells a different story: by controlling glucose, building muscle, and aligning with your hormones, you can transform your body—and your future—at any age.

Inside you'll discover:

- The **Glucose Blueprint Framework** for stabilizing blood sugar and unlocking fat burning
- A fat loss meal timing system that lowers cortisol, improves insulin sensitivity, and burns fat overnight and more.

This is not a diet. It's not about restriction.
It's about **reinvention**—learning how to eat, train, and live in a way that works *with* your body, not against it.

Stronger muscles. Balanced hormones. Steady energy. Sustainable fat loss.

It's time to stop chasing diets and start building *your blueprint for transformation.*

"Finally, a science-backed, women-focused roadmap for lasting fat loss and body transformation."

References

https://pmc.ncbi.nlm.nih.gov/articles/PMC5161655/
https://journals.plos.org/plosone/article?id=10.1371%2Fjournal.pone.0284216
https://www.sciencedirect.com/science/article/abs/pii/S016749432400150X
https://pmc.ncbi.nlm.nih.gov/articles/PMC8308821/
https://www.uchealth.org/today/what-women-need-to-know-about-strength-training/
https://pmc.ncbi.nlm.nih.gov/articles/PMC6719123/
https://pmc.ncbi.nlm.nih.gov/articles/PMC9992880/
https://pmc.ncbi.nlm.nih.gov/articles/PMC7674895/
https://pmc.ncbi.nlm.nih.gov/articles/PMC9986487/
https://www.news-medical.net/news/20250930/Study-shows-prediabetes-remission-does-not-always-require-weight-loss.aspx
https://www.nature.com/articles/s41366-025-01726-4
https://www.nature.com/articles/s41591-025-03944-9
https://www.health.harvard.edu/blog/low-carb-diet-helps-cut-blood-sugar-levels-in-people-with-prediabetes-202301032869
https://www.nature.com/articles/s41366-025-01726-4
https://www.news-medical.net/news/20250930/Study-shows-prediabetes-remission-does-not-always-require-weight-loss.aspx
https://pubmed.ncbi.nlm.nih.gov/37661106/
https://www.sciencedirect.com/science/article/pii/S2667368124000299
https://pubmed.ncbi.nlm.nih.gov/39892489/
https://www.ncbi.nlm.nih.gov/books/NBK572151/
https://www.nature.com/articles/s41392-024-01931-z
https://www.ncbi.nlm.nih.gov/books/NBK572151/

https://pubmed.ncbi.nlm.nih.gov/39892489/
https://pmc.ncbi.nlm.nih.gov/articles/PMC8189979/
https://www.nature.com/articles/nutd201731
https://www.sciencedirect.com/science/article/abs/pii/
S074937971100465X

Summary of References

The provided sources examine various aspects of **metabolic health, weight management, and physical fitness interventions.**

Several texts discuss the **Glucagon-Like Peptide-1 Receptor Agonists (GLP-1RAs),** detailing their mechanisms in regulating glucose and appetite, their effectiveness for weight loss, and their broad therapeutic potential across multiple body systems, including cardiovascular, nervous, and musculoskeletal systems.

Other research focuses on the impact of **lifestyle interventions** like calorie restriction (CR) and exercise (EX), reporting on the undesirable loss of lean mass and bone density often associated with CR alone, while another study concludes that **prediabetes remission** can be achieved without weight loss through improved insulin sensitivity and GLP-1 function.

Finally, one source highlights the benefits of **strength training for women**, emphasizing its role in preserving muscle and bone density as they age, while a meta-analysis specifically compares muscle strength gains in the upper and lower body from resistance training.

www.ingramcontent.com/pod-product-compliance
Lightning Source LLC
Chambersburg PA
CBHW070552270326
41926CB00013B/2282